Coping with Crohn's and Colitis

This practical guide provides patients who have inflammatory bowel disease (IBD) with cognitive-behavioral therapy (CBT) strategies for coping with IBD. It teaches a number of skills that can make coping with Crohn's or colitis easier.

Chapters provide an overview of Crohn's and colitis as well as the interplay between stress and the gut, before offering strategies on relaxation training, physical activity, managing stress and avoidance, diet and nutrition, and medical treatment options. The book also emphasizes the importance of the doctor-patient relationship and helps patients learn how to think about medical management (including the possibility of surgery) to minimize anxiety from catastrophic thoughts and balance potential risks and benefits appropriately. Dr. Hunt challenges readers to engage in specific behavioral experiments to reduce shame and stigma and highlights practical applications with case illustrations and clinical vignettes.

This book can be used as a standalone self-help book or in conjunction with practitioners during in-person therapy.

Melissa G. Hunt is a psychologist, therapist and clinical scientist who specializes in helping folks with chronic GI disorders reclaim their lives.

"Dr. Hunt's book on coping with IBD is timely. The emotional health of patients with Crohn's and ulcerative colitis is often neglected, but so critical to living well with IBD. This book can empower patients to take control of how they think, feel and behave around their symptoms and the settings in which they occur."

Laurie Keefer, PhD, *GI Psychologist and Professor of Medicine and Psychiatry, Icahn School of Medicine at Mount Sinai, New York City*

"Dr. Hunt has done a masterful job in authoring this treatment guide. It provides a toolbox for patients and caregivers alike to be able to understand and address challenges in daily living that may arise in individuals plagued with inflammatory bowel disease, leading to substantially improved quality of life."

Gary R. Lichtenstein, MD, FACG, FACP, AGAF; *Professor of Medicine, Raymond and Ruth Perelman School of Medicine, University of Pennsylvania; Director, Center for Inflammatory Bowel Disease, Department of Medicine, Division of Gastroenterology, University of Pennsylvania Health System.*

Coping with Crohn's and Colitis

A Patient and Clinician's Guide to CBT for IBD

Melissa G. Hunt

Foreword by Aaron T. Beck

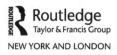
Routledge
Taylor & Francis Group

NEW YORK AND LONDON

First published 2022
by Routledge
605 Third Avenue, New York, NY 10158

and by Routledge
2 Park Square, Milton Park, Abingdon, Oxon OX14 4RN

Routledge is an imprint of the Taylor & Francis Group, an informa business

© 2022 Melissa G. Hunt

Library of Congress Cataloging-in-Publication Data
A catalog record for this title has been requested

ISBN: 978-0-367-52374-9 (hbk)
ISBN: 978-0-367-52367-1 (pbk)
ISBN: 978-1-003-05763-5 (ebk)

DOI: 10.4324/9781003057635

Typeset in Bembo
by Taylor & Francis Books

This book is dedicated to the many IBD patients it has been my privilege to work with over the last ten years. From IBD list-serves and folks who were participants in my early studies, to folks I met at CCF support groups, to a few generous stakeholders who provided me with feedback on early versions of this book, and especially to the folks I have seen in my private practice, I hope you know I learned at least as much, if not more, from you as you ever did from me. It has been my honor to help you cope with Crohn's or colitis.

Contents

About the Author

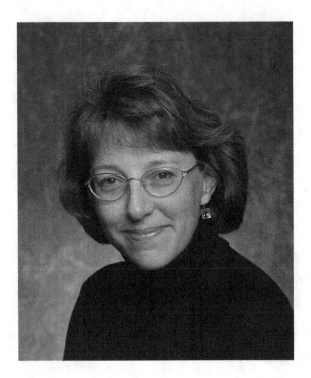

Figure 0.1

My name is Melissa G. Hunt and I'm a licensed clinical psychologist who specializes in cognitive-behavioral therapy (CBT). I serve as the Associate Director of Clinical Training in the Department of Psychology at the University of Pennsylvania. I am very fortunate to be able to combine teaching, supervising young clinicians, doing research and seeing patients. Each aspect of my professional life informs the others. I know that seeing patients makes me a better scientist, and doing research makes me a more effective therapist.

I am always amazed that distressed people entrust me with their personal stories and are willing to share their pain in hopes that they may be able to feel better and to live richer, more productive and more joyful lives. I am always thrilled when basic and applied science can be brought to bear to improve our treatments and help people feel better.

This workbook grew directly out of my experiences working with a number of patients with gut problems in my private practice. This workbook is also the result of 20 years I have spent engaged in the study and investigation of cognitive-behavioral approaches to understanding depression, anxiety, life stress and behavioral health. CBT is a very problem-focused, practical approach to managing life's difficulties. It is also strongly grounded in science. That means the interventions you see here grew out of basic scientific principles. It *also* means that CBT has been tested in literally hundreds of scientific studies. Each study that is done helps us to determine whether or not a treatment approach is actually helpful to people with a particular problem. Treatment studies also help us understand *how* and *why* a particular set of interventions may be helpful.

I am extraordinarily grateful to the many patients I have worked with over the last two decades. Their courage, hope, resilience, insight and willingness to work never fail to inspire me.

Pain is inevitable. Suffering is optional.

Anonymous

Foreword

It has now been 40 years since I published *Cognitive Therapy and the Emotional Disorders* and I continue to be delighted that practitioners of cognitive-behavioral therapy keep expanding the range of disorders this therapy can be applied to. Cognitive-behavioral therapy, or CBT, was a truly revolutionary approach in its day. I was initially trained in psychoanalysis. However, as I used this psychoanalytic approach with my clients, I found that many of the pertinent and most salient statements made by the clients regarded their thoughts, beliefs and general outlooks. Realizing these elements held importance, I began to ask clients about these beliefs and cognitive patterns, which very quickly led to a lessening of symptoms. Unlike earlier models of personality and psychopathology, which assumed that people were essentially irrational and motivated to be self-destructive, cognitive therapy started with the assumption that people were basically rational and were motivated to be healthy and well. Unfortunately, people sometimes developed beliefs that were incorrect, or experienced systematic bias in the way they interpreted their experiences that led them to behave in ways that didn't serve them well and left them more distressed and impaired than was necessary for adaptive functioning. Cognitive theory and therapy, together with advances in learning theory and behavior therapy, soon became a complete system of psychotherapy. CBT is inherently optimistic, respectful and collaborative. In addition, CBT is based in science. First, the therapeutic strategies need to be drawn directly from scientific theory and principles. Second, solid evidence based on randomized controlled trials must support the efficacy of the approach – that is, to prove that it is actually helpful to people. This book exemplifies both of these fundamental attributes of CBT.

Since my early work in the field developing cognitive therapy for depression, CBT has been applied successfully to a wide array of psychological disorders, including anxiety disorders, obsessive-compulsive disorder, post-traumatic stress disorder, borderline personality disorder and schizophrenia. CBT has also been successfully applied to a range of medical disorders that have central nervous system processing as a core part of their etiology, including chronic pain, fibromyalgia and irritable bowel syndrome. There is, of course, a wide range of biologically based diseases and disorders that cognitive-behavioral therapy cannot *cure*. However, even in these instances, CBT can certainly *help* in managing stress, identifying unhelpful or catastrophic beliefs, and building adaptive coping and problem-solving skills. Conditions like cancer, diabetes and a variety of autoimmune disorders including the inflammatory bowel diseases (IBDs) present unique challenges in living. Secondary depression and anxiety, which may arise in part from negative thought patterns and behavioral avoidance, can make those conditions even harder to live with. Fortunately, CBT has been shown to improve quality of life and to reduce depression and anxiety in individuals struggling with IBDs. Unfortunately, finding a trained and certified cognitive-behavioral therapist who has expertise in treating those with gastrointestinal (GI) disorders can be extremely difficult or impossible for many clients. This lack of expertise in both CBT and GI disorders in the therapist and inaccessibility to this treatment demonstrate a clear gap in the field and a crucial need for the existence of this volume. For these reasons among others, I am so pleased that Dr. Melissa Hunt has written this book. Dr. Hunt is recognized broadly as a highly qualified cognitive-behavioral therapist, researcher, teacher and administrator. Dr. Hunt also has a deep understanding of GI disorders and has considerable experience working directly with individuals with GI disorders.

The treatment outlined in this book is not a panacea, but it will be a helping and healing tool. Dr. Hunt will help you learn to manage stress effectively so it does not exacerbate your condition. She will support you in overcoming the shame and secrecy that so often accompany IBDs and isolate you from people you work with and those you love. She will teach you how to counter any catastrophic negative beliefs you might hold that make you feel worse about yourself, your situation or your future. She will gently guide you to figure out how to reduce avoiding recreational, occupational and social opportunities based on anxiety or fear about your IBD symptoms. Importantly, this book provides a wealth of information about how to understand your IBD and your treatment options, including information on how to manage your symptoms proactively with your gastroenterologist. In sum, this book uses expert, GI informed CBT to help you *cope* with the many challenges of living with an IBD, gain a more positive outlook and build resiliency when symptoms, related emotions or thought patterns become very difficult to overcome.

While this book truly delivers in helping clients in all of the ways mentioned above and more, the research that gives credence to this book's efficacy only adds to the confidence and excitement I have about this book. Dr. Hunt tested the efficacy of this book in a randomized controlled trial and the results were uplifting to say the least. In the trial, IBD patients who read the book showed significant decreases in depression and anxiety and experienced greatly improved health-related quality of life that persisted over time. These research findings illuminate both the high-quality content found in this book and the real sense of hope and well-being that this therapy instills in those who read it. We are fortunate that Dr. Hunt has made exceptional cognitive-behavioral therapy available to anyone living with an IBD who wishes to improve his or her quality of life. Dr. Hunt has truly succeeded in taking the core scientific principles and treatment strategies that comprise CBT and applying them specifically to the experience of living with an IBD. This volume is an essential resource for those living with IBDs, their family members and professionals in the psychology and gastroenterology fields alike.

Aaron T. Beck, M.D.
University Professor Emeritus of Psychiatry
University of Pennsylvania
Perelman School of Medicine

Introduction

How to Use This Book – Patients

This book is meant to be a self-help workbook. What does that mean exactly? First, it means you will be working through it *yourself*. That means it's up to you to read the book, at your own pace, and think about how it applies to you. It also means that using this book will take some *work*. That is, you can't just read it (and not do any of the exercises in it) and expect it to do you any good. Chances are that if you're reading this, your inflammatory bowel disease (IBD) and gastro-intestinal (GI) symptoms are interfering with your life and causing you a good deal of distress, and you're probably looking for a better way to cope and manage the day-to-day challenges of living with an IBD. I think this book will help.

I've done my best to fill the book with clinical examples, at least some of which will hopefully capture some of your experiences. I've tried to put enough anecdotes and sample thought records and behavioral experiments (many of them from the real-life experiences of patients with IBDs) for each type of exercise and assignment that it shouldn't be hard to figure out how to apply them to your unique situation. I suggest that you give yourself a timetable for working through the book. If you're fairly consistent, it should take about six weeks to work through the whole thing. Ideally, you'll be able to follow the schedule below more or less. Of course, in the real world, holidays, or travel, or family obligations or work deadlines intervene, so don't worry about it if it's not convenient or possible to do it exactly this way. But do try not to get too behind schedule. I find that it's helpful to get some momentum going with these things, and the chapters do build on each other. On the other hand, don't try to work through it all too quickly either. You need some time to think about the material and practice the various skills and exercises outlined in the book. If you try to go to fast, you won't have a chance to apply things in the real world. You have to let enough "life" happen between chapters to see how the new ways of thinking and approaching things can change your outlook and the way you manage things.

Suggested Schedule

Week 1 – Read Chapters 1–3 and start practicing the relaxation exercises in Chapter 3.

DOI: 10.4324/9781003057635-1

Week 2 – Read Chapter 4 and start trying to do thought records.

Week 3 – Read Chapter 5 and start applying the thought record technique to your GI symptoms.

Week 4 – Read Chapter 6 and think of some behavioral experiments to try.

Week 5 – Read Chapter 7 and think about any avoidance behaviors you could tackle with some exposure therapy.

Week 6 – Read Chapters 8 and 9 to think about how diet, nutrition, healthy choices, medication and even surgery can all play a positive, helpful role in managing your IBD and improving your quality of life. If you have an ostomy, or your doctor has advised that you consider it, or if you just live in fear that you might need one someday, read Chapter 10 as well.

Week 7 through the rest of your life – Read Chapter 11 and review everything you've thought about and tried in the preceding weeks. Continue to practice the skills you've learned, applying them to each new situation and time period in your life. The wonderful thing about the skills taught in this book is that once you get them, you never forget them, and as long as you use them, they will continue to help.

Of course, no self-help book can possibly take the place of good medical care. I strongly urge you to consult with your gastroenterologist and/or internist before making any changes to your diet or medication regimen. You should, of course, follow your doctor's guidance. If your doctor recommends something that doesn't make sense to you, be sure to ask for a good explanation. Don't be shy about this! *You* are the most important member of your treatment team.

How to Use This Book – Clinicians

There are several kinds of clinicians who might be interested in using this book to facilitate patient care.

Gastroenterologists are highly skilled and knowledgeable about the diagnosis and medical management of inflammatory bowel diseases. But you may be less comfortable managing psychiatric co-morbidities like depression or agoraphobia. Moreover, even the most compassionate and humane GI doc simply won't have time to attend to all the many emotional and lifestyle issues that arise for IBD patients. Even if you are fortunate enough to have a dedicated clinical psychologist working in your clinic, who is familiar with GI issues and can practice from an integrative behavioral health perspective, that individual may be overwhelmed with consults. And of course, most GI clinics don't have such an in-house person to manage the emotional and behavioral support piece. This book can help to fill that gap. Having the book available to recommend or to give to patients can be an easy way to provide them with evidence-based support.

There is strong evidence for the value of adding psychological interventions to standard medical care for IBD (Sajadinejad et al., 2012; Szigethy et al., 2017). Indeed, most international guidelines for the management of IBD call for attention to psychosocial issues and psychological distress (Häuser et al.,

2014). Unfortunately, the psychological sequelae and co-morbidities of IBD often remain untreated (Evertsz', Bockting et al., 2012; Evertsz', Thijssens et al., 2012). Despite this, many patients with IBD *desire* psychotherapy and per-ceive it as helpful, but there is a significant gap between their desire for mental health treatment and their actual interactions with providers. Cost and the dearth of IBD-knowledgeable therapists have been identified as the primary barriers to care (Craven, Quinton & Taft, 2018). So one of the best ways to present this book to patients is to acknowledge that being diagnosed with an IBD can be upsetting, and that learning to live with an IBD can be challenging and may take some adjustment on their part. Let patients know that you take their emotional well-being seriously, and that this book has been proven to help with coping with an IBD, so that people can have better quality of life.

Nurse specialists and nurse practitioners in gastroenterology often have dual roles in providing both medical evaluation and care *and* in providing counseling for health and education for patients (e.g. Mayberry & Mayberry, 2003). Indeed, patients with IBD perceive specialist nurses as being particularly able to provide support, advice, caring and empathy as well as information about dis-ease management (Belling, Woods & McLaren, 2008). This book can serve as an important adjunct to the personalized care nurses provide. Indeed, in the UK, nurse supported, low intensity CBT has proven to be quite helpful to GI patients (Dainty et al., 2017). Nurses often have their fingers on the pulse of a patient's health-related quality of life, and can suggest this book to any patient who seems to be struggling with adjustment, or with depression or anxiety. Try presenting the book in a neutral way, by saying, "Many other IBD patients have found the tips and strategies in this book to be very helpful." Nurses are often uniquely positioned to begin to address a patient's emotional distress. Beyond your caring, expert support and advice around medical management, this book can provide your patients with more concrete, evidence-based strategies for improving their quality of life.

Psychologists, social workers and counselors well versed in psychogas-troenterology may be very familiar with *all* the concepts in this book. Nevertheless, they may find the book helpful to share with patients, and can certainly use the questionnaires in the book to help evaluate targets of change and treatment response.

Psychologists, social workers and counselors who are very well trained in evidence-based and empirically supported treatments like cognitive-behavioral therapy may have little knowledge about or experience working with patients with IBDs. A mental health professional with basic comfort with CBT will find much in the structure and format of this approach that feels very familiar. Reading the book in advance of working with an IBD patient will help you "fill in the blanks" in your knowledge. You may be an expert at helping patients learn to do thought records, but the specific cognitive distortions and fears many patients with IBD have may be totally new to you. Getting the lay of the land with these complex GI disorders and understanding the concerns your patients *may* be likely to have can facilitate your work. For example, bowel control anxiety (fear of fecal incontinence) can result in agoraphobia. The very real potential adverse effects of some medications for IBD can contribute to emotional reactivity (e.g. steroids) or feed health anxiety about liver failure or cancer. Fatigue and joint pain can make exercise difficult and can contribute to demoralization and depression. It really *is* hard to talk to friends and colleagues about GI issues, which can worsen social anxiety and isolation. So you can read this book on your own to gain knowledge about this particular population, and use the text as a treatment "manual" to inform your work. Appendix D contains two sample treatment protocols that illustrate the CBT approach with two very different (hypothetical) patients, one with recent onset ulcerative colitis (UC) and the other with long standing Crohn's Disease.

You can also use the book with patients as adjunctive bibliotherapy. Patients can work through each chapter, and you can provide extra support, clarification and correction. For example, the book has a section on teaching deep diaphragmatic breathing (DDB) that most patients can benefit from. But nothing beats being in the room with a clinician who can help pace the breathing and correct the technique if the patient is engaging in shallow thoracic breathing by mistake. And you can remind your patient that done properly, DDB optimizes intestinal motility! The book has many clinical examples that patients can use to learn the basic thought record technique. But many patients can use help and direction in learning to distinguish the objective situation from their thoughts and appraisals from their feelings and subsequent behaviors. Moreover, some patients get "stuck" and can't think of benign alternatives to their catastrophic beliefs. Finally, coming up with graded exposures sometimes takes real creativity and a willingness to carve things up into manageable chunks. This is where a skilled therapist can play an important role, especially if they are somewhat knowledgeable about the GI issues the patient is coping with. So have the patient work through each section of the book and have them practice relaxation exercises or complete thought records or exposures for homework, and then review those experiences with them in the next session.

Psychologists, social workers, counselors and other mental health professionals without much experience in CBT can still use this book as a treatment manual or as adjunctive bibliotherapy with their patients with IBD. The book spells out the basic CBT approach in straightforward modules. Indeed, some of the chapters (like Chapter 4) are really a primer on basic CBT concepts and intervention strategies. You and your patient can work through the book together. You may be surprised by the power and richness of the CBT approach, not just for patients with IBD, but for patients with other issues as well.

In sum, this book can serve as a way for busy gastroenterologists to acknowledge and address the emotional needs of their patients, it can work as a standalone self-help treatment for patients to work through on their own, as adjunctive bibliotherapy to use with the help of a guiding clinician, or as a treatment manual that mental health professionals can use to learn how to do CBT for patients with IBDs.

No matter who you are, I hope you find this book helpful.

Legal Caveats

The information in this book is solely the opinion of Melissa Hunt, Ph.D. and is not intended to replace any recommendations or treatments you are currently receiving from your health care providers.

This book does not exist to provide mental health treatment and should never be used for any crisis situations. If you are suffering from an anxiety disorder, depression or some other problem you should seek treatment from a trained and licensed mental health provider, such as a clinical psychologist, psychiatrist or licensed clinical social worker. If you are in need of immediate care, please call 911 or go to your nearest emergency room.

We are not responsible for damages of any kind arising from use of the book, or from any information contained therein.

No patient/therapist relationship is implied or actualized through the book or through contact with Dr. Hunt about the book.

We may provide links to other resources. We do not thoroughly check linked websites for accuracy or investigate claims made on other linked sites. We are not responsible for the accuracy of any content published on any other linked site. Links provided are not an endorsement of any site or other third-party service.

1   Understanding Crohn's and Colitis

Susannah is a 24-year-old woman who is working towards her Master's degree in elementary education and student teaching in a local school system. Bright, hard-working, warm and creative, she loves working with the kids and she has gotten great feedback from her mentor teacher and the school principal. But Susannah has developed an awful, embarrassing problem that she works hard to keep secret from her co-workers and from her students. She suffers from frequent bouts of burning abdominal pain and diarrhea when the urge to defecate comes on her so suddenly and powerfully, she is never sure she'll make it to the bathroom on time. It's manageable when it happens at home and she can simply run to the bathroom. But she fears having an attack when she is working with the kids at school or when she is trapped in a class in her Master's program. She knows stress often makes it worse, and some foods seem to exacerbate her symptoms too. She's been to the doctor numerous times. First, he recommended that she eat more fiber. That made her symptoms worse. Then he recommended using anti-diarrheal medications like Imodium. That helped a little, but eventually the pain and diarrhea came back, accompanied by occasional mucous and blood in her stools. She started to feel fatigued, her joints started to hurt and she stopped running – an activity she used to love. Despite not exercising as much, she lost some weight. It was hard to put back on since she wasn't very hungry and had started to be afraid of the pain that might follow eating. Her doctor shrugged his shoulders and told her she probably had irritable bowel syndrome and that there wasn't much that could be done except avoiding stress or trying various elimination diets, like limiting gluten or dairy. One night, she woke up in so much pain her fiancé insisted on taking her to the ER. They couldn't find anything wrong, but they did refer her to a gastroenterologist. The new doctor ran a number of tests and discovered that Susannah was anemic and deficient in several important vitamins, including B12. He also found blood in her stool, and inflammatory markers in her stool and blood. The gastroenterologist had her schedule an MRE (magnetic resonance enterography) and a colonoscopy. A week later, after all that testing, she finally had a diagnosis: ulcerative colitis. It was nice to know what was actually wrong, but now she wonders if she will ever be able to finish her program, much less work full time as a teacher. She is devastated by the diagnosis, fearful of the long-term implications and is thinking about breaking things off with her fiancé. Suddenly the happy, fulfilling, productive life she envisioned for herself just doesn't seem possible anymore.

DOI: 10.4324/9781003057635-2

Mike is a 54-year-old regional sales manager for a major consumer products company. He was diagnosed with Crohn's Disease when he was 14 and has been living with it ever since. He's married and has two kids and a full-time job. But he keeps his Crohn's Disease secret from everyone but his wife. He just assumes that people would be disgusted and repulsed by him if they knew what he dealt with. He also assumes that his boss and his team would question his competence and his ability to manage the rigors of his job. Because his job involves frequent travel and long meetings, he has invented all sorts of excuses and stories to explain his occasional absence or disappearance. He doesn't drink and is pretty careful to manage his diet, so meeting with a sales team or client over dinner or in a hotel bar just doesn't work. In fact, he never eats at work functions, and when he's having a flare, he always excuses himself and retires to his hotel room. His go-to excuse is that he ate a "bad burrito" at the airport. He's ashamed of his gut problems and believes it would be humiliating if anyone found out. Even when his gastroenterologist assures him that he's in remission, he's vigilant about monitoring his GI symptoms and eats a very restrictive, low residue, low FODMAP diet just to be "on the safe side." In fact, he often experiences visceral (or gut) pain and alternating diarrhea and constipation when he's supposed to be in remission, and he wonders if his doctor is missing something. He worries a lot about the implications of his disease for his job. While his wife is quietly sympathetic, his kids sometimes tease their dad about his long "bathroom breaks" and his "weird" bland diet. This makes him angry and frustrated, but he doesn't know what to do about it. He also typically avoids going to his son's soccer and baseball games and tournaments and his daughter's gymnastics and swimming meets, even when he is in town, because it's just too hard to find a bathroom in those settings. He feels increasingly alienated from his kids but can't figure out what to do about that either. Still, he lives in fear of someone finding out about his "bathroom issues" and will go to any lengths to keep this shameful secret from leaking out. He lives in terror of being told he needs an ostomy. He can't imagine how he would cope if that happened.

People who are living with inflammatory bowel diseases have many different experiences and everyone's individual story is unique. Some people seem to just shrug off the diagnosis. They manage the disease with the help of a good gastroenterologist and just go about their lives. But if you're like many people with an inflammatory bowel disease (IBD), you may find something in these stories that feels familiar. You may also want *someone* to help you figure out how to minimize the impact of your IBD on your well-being and your ability to live life to the fullest. Gastroenterologists who specialize in IBDs like Crohn's and ulcerative colitis are absolutely the experts when it comes to the *medical* management of your disease. They are the ones who can perform needed diagnostic procedures and will recommend dietary modifications, medications and occasionally surgical interventions to treat the biological aspects of IBDs. But GI doctors *don't* typically specialize in helping you think about the emotional and practical side of living with an IBD – that is, how to *cope*. Doctors may suggest that you try to "avoid stress" but that is neither helpful nor possible in the real world. Nor do GI docs or specialized nurses have time to help you think through what to tell your in-laws or your boss or your clients about your condition and the things you have to do to manage it effectively. GI docs can answer specific questions you have about the side effects of medications or the likelihood that you'll require surgery, but they are not trained to help you manage any anxiety, frustration, depression or embarrassment you might be experiencing. Living with an inflammatory bowel disease can be challenging, but it need not keep you from living a full life.

This book was written to address all these *other* aspects of living with an inflammatory bowel disease. If Crohn's or ulcerative colitis is robbing you of productive work, satisfying relationships or joyful play, then it is time to reclaim your life.

First, let's acknowledge that it can often take a long time to get a correct diagnosis. Many individuals who are ultimately diagnosed with an IBD spend months or even *years* in considerable discomfort and ill health before a doctor finally figures out what's going on. Many individuals endure multiple hospitalizations and *wrong* diagnoses before getting a correct diagnosis. Many individuals with IBDs have at some point been tested for lactose intolerance and Celiac Disease, and may have tried various elimination diets (limiting lactose-rich milk products or gluten or meat or legumes or eggs or fruits or sugars or fat or spicy food or alcohol or caffeine or… the list is almost endless). Probably the most frustrating wrong diagnosis is irritable bowel syndrome (or IBS). IBS is typically diagnosed based on the clinical symptoms of recurrent abdominal pain (typically relieved by defecation), accompanied by a change in the form or frequency of stool. IBS can result in chronic constipation, chronic diarrhea or an alternating mix of the two. Since abdominal pain and frequent diarrhea are also the hallmark symptoms of inflammatory bowel diseases, it's easy to see how the different conditions could be confused.

The first indication a doctor should look for that might suggest something other than IBS is a collection of so-called "alarm" symptoms. These are all things that suggest an underlying inflammatory or infectious process. Alarm symptoms include fever, elevated inflammatory markers in your blood work, anemia or other nutritional deficiencies (which suggest malabsorption of nutrients by a compromised intestine), blood in your stools (which might suggest ulcerations, an abscess or fistula), and pain that wakes you up from a sound sleep. To make a positive diagnosis of Crohn's or ulcerative colitis, your gastroenterologist will generally need to actually take a look at your intestines and take small samples of tissue to confirm the inflammatory process.

Crohn's Disease is an inflammatory bowel disease that can cause abdominal pain and diarrhea. Crohn's Disease can also cause rectal bleeding, weight loss, ulcers in the intestines, arthritis, skin problems, and fever. Sometimes the bleeding is serious enough that it leads to anemia, and people may develop malnutrition as the inflammation of the lining of the intestines worsens. Crohn's Disease can also cause ulcers or sores in other parts of the body, including the esophagus, the throat and the mouth. The inflammation spans the entire thickness of the intestinal wall (technically called transmural inflammation). Sometimes the intestines actually become blocked by thickened scar tissue that is the result of long-term inflammation. This can be a life-threatening emergency that requires immediate medical care.

Crohn's Disease is almost certainly an autoimmune disorder in which the body's immune system starts to attack both helpful (symbiotic) bacteria that normally live in the gut and gut tissue itself. This chronic inflammatory response causes damage to the digestive tract, which can result in ulcers, thickened scar tissue, tears, bleeding and malnutrition, including anemia secondary to blood loss and more general nutritional deficits due to malabsorption of food.

To diagnose Crohn's Disease, your doctor will check for a number of things. Using blood tests, they will check your complete blood count (CBC), sedimentation rate and C-reactive protein, all of which might reveal underlying inflammation. They will also check your hemoglobin and vitamin B12 levels. Some people with Crohn's will show signs of anemia, which can suggest that ulcers in the intestines are causing bleeding and/or that they are not absorbing sufficient iron from their food. B12 deficiencies are also common because B12 is absorbed by the ileum (the last section of the small intestine) which is a very common location for Crohn's inflammation. In addition to blood work, the doctor will probably also ask you to take small stool samples for several days, and will check those samples for blood (called a fecal occult blood test), which can also suggest bleeding in the intestines. He or she will probably also order a fecal calprotectin test, which can be done with a larger stool sample. Calprotectin is a marker of inflammation specifically in the intestines. It's very sensitive and can be used both diagnostically (to distinguish an IBD from IBS) and to track disease severity in an IBD.

Ultimately, your doctor will want to get a good look at your intestines. There are a number of ways to do this. In an upper GI and small bowel series or CT scan you will need to drink barium, a slightly sweet, chalky white liquid that coats the lining of the small intestine, making it easier to see what's going on. After drinking the barium, you will have X-rays or a CT scan taken. The barium looks white in the images, and shows spots where there may be inflammation or other abnormalities in the small intestine. In a lower GI series, you will have to take barium in the form of an enema, which will be administered by the doctor. Then X-rays or CT scans are taken of your large intestines, including the colon and rectum.

While many doctors and hospitals still use these tried and true procedures, a newer way to visualize the intestines is with MRE (magnetic resonance enterography). MRE is more sensitive to real time changes than CT scans are, so it's able to tell the difference between a narrowing that's due to normal peristalsis (muscle contractions that move food along) and a narrowing that's due to a stricture, or the formation of scar tissue.

Another way to get a look at your intestines is for the doctor to do an actual visual exam by performing a sigmoidoscopy, a colonoscopy or a capsule endoscopy. In both a sigmoidoscopy and a colonoscopy, the doctor inserts a flexible lighted tube into the anus and up through part of the large intestine. Flexible sigmoidoscopy lets the doctor see only the last third of the large intestine (the sigmoid colon). Colonoscopy allows the doctor to see the *entire* large intestine, and *sometimes* the terminal ileum (or the last bit of the small intestine) so it's usually the better procedure, although it does take a bit more time and effort to prepare for it. In both cases, the scope transmits images of the lining of the intestine to a computer or video monitor. The doctor can actually *see* if there is any inflammation, ulcers or bleeding. Both procedures also allow the doctor to remove any polyps or other growths and to take very small samples of tissue or biopsies, which can then be looked at carefully under a microscope.

It's very difficult for doctors to get physical scopes with cameras and biopsy tools into most of the small intestine, and it's important to get a look at it, since Crohn's Disease activity is sometimes confined to the small intestine. The best way to visualize the entire small intestine is with a capsule endoscopy. In this amazing procedure, you swallow a tiny camera that is safely inside a capsule no bigger than the average vitamin pill. As it travels through the GI tract, it transmits multiple pictures to a small receiver worn on a belt. The capsule is disposable and passes out of your system with a bowel movement. (You don't have to worry about trying to retrieve it!) The advantage of this is that it lets your doctor see the *entire* small intestine. The disadvantage is that there's no way to take tissue samples, so there are no biopsies to analyze. But all of these procedures allow the doctor to actually *see* if there is any inflammation, ulcers, fistulas, strictures or other signs of Crohn's.

Ulcerative colitis (UC) is the other main inflammatory bowel disease. UC, like Crohn's Disease, can also cause inflammation and ulcers in the lining of the rectum and colon, but unlike Crohn's Disease the inflammation occurs only in the top layer of the lining of the large intestine. Ulcers can form where inflammation has killed the cells that usually line the colon. Like Crohn's Disease, this can often result in intestinal bleeding, leading to anemia and bloody stools. Like IBS and Crohn's, the most common symptoms of ulcerative colitis are abdominal pain or cramps and frequent diarrhea. Other complications include anemia, weight loss, loss of appetite, fever, skin lesions, joint pain and rectal bleeding. Like Crohn's Disease, UC is thought to result from a disorder of the immune system.

UC is diagnosed in much the same way Crohn's Disease is, with a combination of blood work, analysis of stool samples, and visualization studies. Because UC differs from Crohn's Disease in how deep the inflammation goes in the intestinal wall, the doctor will need to take tissue samples for microscopic analysis to make a definitive diagnosis.

Microscopic colitis (MC) is another form of inflammatory bowel disease. The main symptoms are, of course, watery diarrhea and abdominal pain. There are two types of microscopic colitis – lymphocytic and collagenous. In the collagenous type, a thick layer of protein (or collagen) develops in the tissues of the colon. In the lymphocytic type, white blood cells proliferate in the tissues of the colon. It is not known whether these are truly two different subtypes or two stages of the same inflammatory process. In both cases, the symptom overlap with IBS is considerable. A number of studies have suggested that it is very difficult to distinguish IBS and microscopic colitis on the basis of symptom presentation alone. Indeed, many patients with histologically proven microscopic colitis will also technically meet diagnostic criteria for IBS.

Not surprisingly, MC is also thought to be an autoimmune disorder. Many people with MC also have other autoimmune problems which might include rheumatoid arthritis, psoriasis, Celiac Disease or thyroid problems like Hashimoto's thyroiditis or Graves' disease. In fact, both types of MC show increased white blood cells in the tissues of the colon – and an increased white count is generally a sign of immune system activity or, in this case, over-activity.

A history of having taken certain medications is known to increase the risk for MC. In particular, long-term or chronic use of non-steroidal anti-inflammatory pain killers including aspirin, ibuprofen and naproxen turns out to be very common in people who are ultimately diagnosed with MC. It might seem ironic that using an anti-inflammatory drug would increase the risk of an inflammatory bowel disorder. Unfortunately, this particular class of drugs tends to irritate the lining of the intestines. Oddly, there is a *different* type of anti-inflammatory drug called mesalamine that can be used to treat both ulcerative colitis and microscopic colitis.

Friendly Bacteria or the Human Microbiome

One very intriguing hypothesis about a potential contributing factor in all types of IBDs is that they might be related to disruptions in the human microbiome – that is the population of microorganisms that lives inside us. Throughout most of the history of modern medicine, bacteria have been seen as the enemy. Ever since Louis Pasteur conducted his famous experiments proving that "germs" caused many diseases, the "germ theory" of medicine has held sway. Germ theory turned out to be an incredibly powerful paradigm that shifted medicine away from mostly ineffective and often harmful interventions (like blood-letting) to the successful vanquishing of some of the most virulent and deadly diseases known to man, including smallpox, polio and tuberculosis. The combination of vaccines that teach the immune system to resist viruses and bacteria, and anti-biotics, which actually kill bacterial pathogens, has saved literally hundreds of millions of lives and spared millions more the disfigurement and disability that used to be common hazards for all humans. Germ theory and modern industrial life, with indoor plumbing, clean running water, containment of sewage and safety inspectors in food processing plants, have also dramatically reduced the impact of dangerous bacterial infections like cholera, salmonella and Escherichia (or e.) coli. There is no doubt that germ theory, and the resulting war on germs, has benefited humankind enormously.

But there is a downside to all this anti-germ fervor. There are very good reasons to believe that we have taken this one-sided view of "germs" too far, and are actually now *hurting* ourselves with our endless efforts to disinfect and sterilize our environments. We are constantly advised to wash our hands, disinfect our cutting boards and bathrooms, use hand sanitizers at every opportunity and purchase innumerable products with antimicrobial chemicals embedded in them. This has had three unexpected and quite negative consequences. First, the excessive use of germicidal chemicals has actually spurred the evolution of *resistant super bacteria*. Over-prescription of antibiotics was routine medical practice for years. Only very recently have physicians, researchers, and medical organizations sounded the alarm about the rise of resistant strains of tuberculosis and other frightening bacteria like MRSA (methicillin-resistant Staphylococcus aureus). Indeed, the American Medical Association has issued a position statement warning *against* the use of antimicrobial agents like triclosan in consumer products such as hand sanitizer, dishwashing soap and cutting boards. They cite evidence suggesting that such use is actually *harmful* to public health, because it spurs the development of resistant bacteria.

But even more important for our purposes are the *other* unintended consequences of too much sterilization of our environment. First, those of us who live in the industrialized world are ending up with *dumb immune systems*. There is considerable evidence for the "hygiene hypothesis" that explains the dramatic rise in the incidence of a variety of autoimmune disorders in the developed world, including the IBDs. It turns out that exposure to a wide range of microorganisms before age five is crucial to the development of the immune system. Parents of young children in daycare may bemoan the many sniffles, coughs and runny noses their kids come home with. But they should take heart in knowing that their kids are *much* less likely to develop asthma or serious allergies by the time they're 15 than kids who stayed home until they started kindergarten. When the immune system doesn't get to learn who the bad guys are and how to fight them, it grows up not being able to distinguish the bad guys from the good guys or even the bad guys from the self. This has led to a dramatic rise in autoimmune disorders including allergies, asthma, lupus, rheumatoid arthritis, and the inflammatory bowel diseases in the developed world. As one gastroenterologist I work with put it, "there's a thin line between dying of cholera and developing Crohn's." The incidence of inflammatory bowel diseases like Crohn's in developing countries in Asia, Africa and South America is *tiny*. [1] Goat herders in Ethiopia *don't* get Crohn's Disease, though they may well have intestinal worms.

Amazingly, there have been a few small but promising clinical trials suggesting that a brief intestinal worm infestation (called "Helminth therapy" after the group of intestinal worms typically used) may actually put Crohn's Disease into remission – normalizing the immune system factors that cause the abnormal inflammatory process. Helminths have immunoregulatory abilities that change the way the host's immune system functions in pretty complicated ways that turn out to be helpful for people with IBDs. [2] There was a larger study that did not demonstrate successful results, which was disappointing, but more trials are underway. We would also need to get past the "yuck" factor for it to become a common treatment for Crohn's. A number of researchers are trying to identify the specific chemical signals helminths use that result in immunosuppression in the host. That could eventually lead to useful medications.

The final unintended consequence of the war on germs is that we may very well be killing off the very bacteria that we need to thrive. This is the most challenging part for most Westerners to accept, but we actually live symbiotically with trillions of bacteria *in our own bodies*. In fact, our bodies are composed of about ten alien microorganisms for every one human cell! Collectively, these microorganisms are referred to as the human microbiome. Interestingly, the vast majority of them live *in the gut*. Known as "gut flora," these microorganisms play a vital role in helping us digest our food, keeping pathogenic bacteria in check, educating the immune system and *reducing* inflammation. Keeping these friendly bacterial populations healthy and in the right balance turns out to be crucial for overall *and* digestive health. Scientists have raised mice from birth in completely sterile environments. Their guts are pristine – no bacteria at all. And the mice are a mess. They're puny, weak and can't digest food properly at all.

There is considerable evidence that the gut flora in people with IBDs are quite different from the gut flora of healthy people. That is, there are imbalances in the ecosystem of the gut. We do know that people with Crohn's are particularly vulnerable to clostridium difficile (C. diff) infection. C. diff is a bacterium that is found in small concentrations in healthy people's GI systems. But when the gut flora are out of balance, C. diff can flourish, causing all kinds of serious difficulties. The usual treatment, of course, according to germ theory, is an aggressive course of a very powerful (and expensive) antibiotic called vancomycin. Unfortunately, that approach often backfires in the long run. Why? Because even if you kill some problematic bacteria, you're probably also killing *good* bacteria, and you've done nothing to re-establish the *balance* of the ecosystem in the gut. Imagine you have a terrible weed infestation in your garden. It's taking over everything and killing off the bulbs and flowers and shrubs you actually want. You could try to spread poison to kill the weeds, and it might work temporarily. But what will you be left with? Big patches of withered weeds and bare dirt. You know what's most likely to grow back in those spots? More weeds! You need to fill your garden with the plants you *want*, or you'll be right back where you started. A healthy garden overflowing with irises and zinnias and daisies and roses and lavender and marigolds and petunias and geraniums and snap dragons (you get the picture) is much more resistant to the occasional weed seed because the plants you want keep the weeds from getting enough dirt, water and sun. Without good, helpful, symbiotic bacteria, to colonize the gut and work with us, killing off "bad" bacteria won't ultimately help.

The most dramatic example of the need for "good" bacteria in the gut comes from transplant surgery. When people with serious bowel problems require transplant surgery, physicians used to take great pains to wash and sterilize the donor intestinal tissue.[3] This makes sense from a germ theory perspective. But it turns out to be a really bad idea. Believe it or not, allowing the donor tissue to retain its natural complement of symbiotic bacteria leads to *much* better outcomes for the recipient.

A natural extension of this has been the development of a truly bizarre *sounding* procedure called "fecal microbiota transplantation" or FMT in which stool from a healthy person is inserted (often via enema) into the intestines of someone struggling with an IBD and/or a serious C. diff infection. After all, poop is actually about 30% bacteria. The outcome data on this procedure are growing and highly encouraging, especially in the case of C. diff infections, and even in C. diff infections in folks with an IBD. Long-term follow ups of these patients have shown a complete restoration of *normal gut flora* many months down the road, and the patients remain symptom free, often after a single treatment. Indeed, FMT is now part of clinical practice guidelines for managing C. diff infections, and many gastroenterologists are recommending it for IBD, although it's not standard clinical practice at this point. We still need larger clinical trials before it becomes a main-stream treatment, but this approach is very promising and may offer long-term relief to people with serious GI problems in years to come.

Other Conditions that Cause GI Symptoms

Chances are high that if you're reading this book these other conditions have all been ruled out, and you *know* you have an inflammatory bowel disease. I list them here on the off chance that you haven't had a thorough diagnostic workup and your physician and you aren't actually 100% positive what is causing your symptoms.

Celiac Disease

Celiac Disease is an autoimmune disorder in which the body is unable to break down gluten, one of the major proteins in wheat, rye and barley. When people with Celiac Disease eat foods containing gluten (like bread and pasta), their immune system treats the gluten as a foreign invader and mounts a huge defensive response. Unfortunately, this results in damage to the wall of the small intestine. The small intestine is lined with villi – tiny, finger-like projections that coat the lining of the small intestine and dramatically increase the surface area available for absorbing nutrients from food. In Celiac Disease, the villi are damaged or even destroyed. The most common symptoms of Celiac Disease are – you guessed it – abdominal pain and diarrhea (and sometimes constipation), although the stools in Celiac Disease are usually pale in color. The second most common symptom in adults is anemia, due to malabsorption of nutrients. Like the inflammatory bowel diseases, Celiac Disease can also manifest itself in other parts of the body, leading to fatigue, joint pain, arthritis, canker sores in the mouth or an itchy rash on the skin. People with Celiac Disease are more likely than people in the general population to develop an IBD, and there is some evidence that people with IBDs have an increased risk of Celiac Disease. This is probably because the disorders are all autoimmune diseases, and share some underlying genetic risks and pathophysiology in the tissues of the gut.

To make a positive diagnosis of Celiac Disease, the doctor will start with blood work. Anemia (especially if it doesn't resolve quickly with iron supplements) is a clue that whatever is going on, it is probably not IBS. One very specific test for Celiac Disease is to look for certain antibodies in the blood. It is very important to continue eating a diet that contains gluten for approximately six weeks before the test. If you are already on a gluten-free diet, the tests will come back negative, even if you really do have Celiac Disease. Celiac Disease is partly genetic, and there is actually a genetic test available to see if you carry the genes for it. If you don't, then you *can't* have Celiac Disease. If you do carry the genes, then you *might* have Celiac Disease.

If your symptoms and blood work (and possibly genetic testing) are consistent with Celiac Disease, the doctor will probably want to do an endoscopy, in which a flexible, thin tube is inserted through the mouth and stomach to reach the small intestine. Remember, the inflammatory bowel diseases typically affect the last part of the small intestine, the large intestine, or colon. Celiac Disease affects the villi in the small intestine. During an endoscopy, like a colonoscopy, the doctor will be able to see the lining of the upper part of the small intestine, and will be able to take tissue samples to confirm whether the villi have been damaged.

While Celiac Disease is sometimes present from childhood, it can be triggered in adulthood by a variety of environmental and physical stressors, including surgery, pregnancy, viral infection or even severe emotional stress. So just because you never had trouble with gluten containing foods earlier in life doesn't necessarily mean you don't have Celiac Disease now. Since people with IBDs are at somewhat heightened risk for developing Celiac Disease, and since Celiac Disease can be managed entirely with dietary changes, it's worth being tested for. The good news is that a gluten-free diet will stop the damage being caused by the Celiac Disease and allow your intestines to heal. Unfortunately, a truly gluten-free diet is tricky to maintain. There is "hidden" gluten in a lot of prepared and restaurant foods. But if you educate yourself about it and commit to it, a gluten-free diet can solve the GI symptoms that are the result of Celiac Disease.

On the other hand, if you *don't* have Celiac Disease, it probably makes no sense at all to avoid gluten, even if you have an IBD. Going "gluten free" is a popular fad right now, and there are new (and very expensive) products showing up on the gluten-free shelves every day. This has been a money-making, marketing bonanza for industrial food companies – replacing "fat free" and "sugar free" as a way to appeal to health conscious but naïve consumers. For people with true Celiac, the availability of gluten-free products has been an incredible blessing. In fact, certain gluten-free products (like special breads and pastas) are tax deductible for people with Celiac Disease because they are a medical necessity. For most people, however, avoiding gluten makes no sense and will not have an impact on GI functioning or overall health. Most human beings have no difficulty digesting this protein. Indeed, barley, wheat, and rye have been important staple foods for a significant proportion of the human population for millennia. Limiting your calories from refined carbohydrates like white bread and pasta may be good for your waistline, but eating a gluten-free diet is totally unnecessary for most of us. Lots of people with an IBD *believe* that they may have a non-celiac gluten sensitivity (NCGS) and some folks absolutely swear that they feel better when they avoid gluten.[4] But there is no serious scientific evidence that avoiding gluten is helpful for people with IBDs unless they *also* have Celiac Disease. In fact, following a gluten-free diet is actually associated with lower psychological well-being and more dysbiosis, but no objective benefits in terms of disease severity.[5] That said, if you *do* have Celiac Disease, you really *must* avoid gluten or you risk long-term pain, malabsorption, nutritional deficiencies, and poor health. So it is definitely worth being tested for Celiac Disease with a blood test.

Lactose Intolerance

Another possible cause of worsening GI symptoms is lactose intolerance. Lactose intolerance occurs when the small intestine stops producing the enzyme lactase, which breaks down the sugar lactose that is found in all kinds of milk. What are the symptoms of lactose intolerance? Abdominal pain, gas, bloating and diarrhea, of course!

Interestingly, all human beings produce the lactase enzyme during the first few years of life, because lactose is found in human milk and is necessary for early development. In most people of the world (especially Asians, Southeast Asians, Native Americans and many Africans), lactase production stops around the time that toddlers would typically be weaned. Interestingly, traditional Asian and Native American cuisines typically contain no milk products, consistent with the fact that folks from those ethnic backgrounds do indeed tend to be lactose-intolerant. People in those cultures found ways to combine legumes (like beans or soybeans) with grains (like corn, rice, or wheat) to make complete proteins and provide full nutrition (and delicious cuisines!).

In many other human populations, however, primarily people from pastoral cultures that developed cow, sheep, and goat herding early on (including some African, most Indian, and most European and Middle Eastern peoples), a genetic mutation occurred that kept the lactase production gene *switched on*. You may have heard that humans shouldn't drink cow's milk because we didn't "evolve" to, but in fact this is incorrect. Extended lactase production mutations occurred independently in different human populations at different times.[6] It was a tremendous advantage under certain environmental circumstances, allowing the introduction of cow, goat, sheep, and even reindeer and yak milk products as major forms of dietary protein. Animal milk is a *fantastic* way to turn otherwise totally indigestible grass into a high-quality, complete, tasty, and versatile protein, so the ability to digest it was strongly selected for in those populations where the mutation arose. This is actually *exactly* how evolution works – a spontaneous genetic mutation arises that confers survival and reproductive advantage and is therefore selected for and passed on to the next generation. So, in fact, lots of humans *did* evolve to drink animal milk. But not *all* people did, so there are indeed some people who are lactose-intolerant. Because cow's milk has become such a major part of the Western diet, actually being lactose-intolerant in America or Europe can be quite problematic.

Lactose intolerance is diagnosed in several ways. First, your doctor may recommend trying an "elimination diet." You stop eating *all* dairy products for several weeks and see if the symptoms go away. Then you reintroduce dairy products and see if the symptoms return. There are a number of problems with this approach. First of all, eliminating a whole class of foods usually means changing your diet in lots of ways – you typically increase something else or add a new food entirely (e.g. soy milk or almond milk). You might be reducing the amount of overall fat in your diet (no more ice cream or cheese, after all). You're probably also paying a lot more attention to what and how you're eating – not eating out as much, cooking more carefully, and so on. So it's really hard to know if any changes in your symptoms were actually due to eliminating food A or to introducing or increasing food(s) B, C or D. Another reason elimination diets are problematic is that when you suddenly stop eating a certain type of food, the helpful, symbiotic bacteria that normally live in your gut and help digest that food may die off. When you reintroduce the food, you may feel symptomatic because you've thrown off your microbiome. So elimination diets are actually *not* a very good way to figure out if a food is causing you problems and are pretty nonspecific from a diagnostic perspective.

A much *better* test is the hydrogen breath test. Undigested lactose is broken down by bacteria in the gut, leading to the production of hydrogen and methane gases, which can be detected in the breath. Eventually, a simple genetic test may be used to identify individuals who are lactose-intolerant, but that is not available in routine clinical practice yet. Because the hydrogen breath test, like the Celiac blood test, is not particularly invasive, it's almost certainly worth doing to rule out the possibility that your symptoms are being caused by lactose intolerance. It's certainly possible to be lactose-intolerant *and* have an inflammatory bowel disease, so it's important to rule out. Note that if you are *not* lactose-intolerant, there is probably very little reason to eliminate dairy from your diet.

Colorectal Cancer

Colorectal cancer (or colon cancer) occurs when cells in the large intestine start to multiply in an out of control way. Usually, the tumors begin as polyps – little bumps or growths inside the lining of the large intestine. Most polyps are benign. They usually don't cause symptoms and are not dangerous. But sometimes, polyps become cancerous over time. The symptoms of colon cancer vary and depend on the location and size of the tumor and whether the cancer has metastasized (or spread) to other parts of the body, such as the liver. If the tumor is close to the anus, there may be a change in bowel habits – either diarrhea or constipation. If the tumor begins to block the flow of stools (called a bowel obstruction) the patient may experience abdominal pain, constipation and vomiting. There may also be evidence of blood in the stools. The single best way to diagnose colon cancer is with a colonoscopy. If caught early, colon cancer is almost always treatable. The American Gastroenterological Association advises people who have no risk factors to be tested starting at age 50, while people with a family history of colon cancer should have their first colonoscopy at age 40, or ten years before the age that the relative got cancer, whichever comes first. If you are struggling with serious GI symptoms, however, a colonoscopy can certainly bring peace of mind if it rules out this potentially fatal disease and may provide definitive diagnosis of something else, like an IBD.

Irritable Bowel Syndrome

Irritable bowel syndrome, or IBS, is a disorder of central (brain) and enteric (gut) pain processing in which the messages between the gut and the brain get distorted and amplified. This results in frequent abdominal pain and changes in defecation (either diarrhea, constipation or an alternating mix of the two) and can also result in extreme fecal urgency, gas, bloating, flatulence, feelings of fullness, difficulty fully evacuating stool, fear of fecal incontinence and, often, lots and lots of distress and frustration. One of the most important underlying mechanisms in IBS is the development of *visceral hypersensitivity*. Basically, patients with IBS feel normal gut sensations that most people would be unaware of, and experience many of those sensations as more painful than healthy controls. Visceral hypersensitivity can be measured objectively with balloon distension (of the gastric fundus, descending colon or rectum) and is clearly correlated with IBS symptom severity. Visceral hypersensitivity leads to a vicious cycle of vigilance, stress, increasing pain, and increasing vigilance. That is, being anxious about and paying attention to visceral sensations exacerbates the underlying hypersensitivity leading to escalating cycles of pain and abnormal defecation.

Can I Have Both IBD and IBS?

For most people who are ultimately diagnosed with an inflammatory bowel disease, the journey to diagnosis is long and harrowing. Many patients have been through the proverbial medical wringer – seeing an average of five different doctors, undergoing an average of eight to nine diagnostic tests, and spending more than a year feeling very ill (with almost half having been hospitalized at least once) before they finally get a positive diagnosis. Just hearing that someone has *finally* figured out what's wrong with you may actually be a relief. In fact, IBD patients are sometimes misdiagnosed with IBS for *years* before someone finally figures out what's really going on.

So what do you make of it if a doctor tells you that your IBD is in remission, but you are still having GI symptoms because *now* you have IBS? Is that even possible? Unfortunately, it is. In fact, some studies suggest that about *half* of IBD patients will experience IBS-like symptoms when the IBD itself is in remission. Put another way, IBD patients are about three times as likely to develop IBS as someone in the general population. This may seem horribly unfair. But the good news is that if this is you, then the suggestions in the rest of this book should help *a lot*.

GI symptoms, even when they have a clear underlying medical cause, can be dramatically exacerbated by stress, for fairly straightforward biological reasons (see Chapter 2). Whatever your doctors are doing medically to manage your IBD, effective stress management, and in particular managing the stress that is the direct result of acute IBD flares and GI symptoms, should still bring substantial relief and make your IBD easier to bear. Moreover, there is emerging evidence that having an IBD itself can *cause* alterations in the way the brain and gut communicate with each other.[7] Dysregulation of this brain-gut axis (technically the central-enteric nervous systems) can exacerbate all kinds of GI symptoms, especially pain regulation and motility. IBS *is* a disorder of gut-brain communication. It's understandable that someone who has been living with an IBD would start paying more attention to visceral, or GI sensations. Sometimes you *have to* because those sensations contain important information about inflammation in the body. But sometimes the brain starts paying too much attention to those sensations, and the volume of the pain signaling from the gut gets turned up too high. That's not helpful or informative at all. Fortunately, the techniques in this book will address that issue as well, and can help turn down pain signaling to help you be more comfortable.

Coping with Crohn's and Colitis

Even if stress played no role whatsoever in exacerbating GI symptoms, you might still want to learn some new strategies for managing stress (and your GI symptoms!) more effectively. Living with an IBD is challenging. People with IBDs have a number of serious and legitimate concerns.

- How can I manage my diet and still get adequate nutrition?
- What will happen if I have to take time off of work or school to deal with flare ups and medical procedures?
- Will I be able to take care of my family when I'm ill?
- Can I still be physically active?
- How will I afford all the out-of-pocket medical expenses associated with my illness?
- Should I tell people about my disorder or keep it secret?
- What will people think if I tell them?
- What if I have a serious reaction to a medication?
- What if I need surgery?

In other words, just having an IBD can be a stressful experience in and of itself. That's one reason it can be so frustrating if a doctor tells you to "avoid stress." Ha! As if that were possible! This book was written to help people with an IBD *cope* with all the challenges a chronic GI condition adds to living your life. In other words, I'm not going to suggest that you *avoid* stress. I'm going to teach you how to *manage* it.

Summary

Inflammatory bowel diseases (including Crohn's and ulcerative colitis and the milder version microscopic colitis) are serious medical conditions that are probably the result of an autoimmune response that is out of control. They are very different from irritable bowel syndrome. They are typically accompanied by alarm signs and symptoms that alert you and your doctor to the underlying inflammatory process. IBDs are typically diagnosed after imaging studies, endoscopy or colonoscopy reveal evidence of inflammation and tissue damage. However, it is possible to develop secondary IBS when your IBD is in remission.

Notes

1 Bernstein, C.N., Fried, M, Krabshuis, J.H. et al. (June 2009). Inflammatory bowel disease: A global perspective. *World Gastroenterology Organisation Global Guidelines*. Downloaded from www.worldgastroenterology.org/guidelines/global-guidelines/inflammatory-bowel -disease-ibd/inflammatory-bowel-disease-ibd-english, August 31, 2015.
2 Abdoli, A. (2019). Therapeutic potential of helminths and helminth-derived antigens for resolution of inflammation in inflammatory bowel disease. *Archives of Medical Research*, https://doi.org/10.1016/j.arcmed.2019.03.001.
3 Kim, K.O. & Gluck, M. (2019). Fecal microbiota transplantation: An update on clinical practice. *Clinical Endoscopy*, 52(2), 137–143.
4 Herfarth, H.H., Martin, C.F., Sandler, R.S. et al. (2014). Prevalence of a gluten-free diet and improvement of clinical symptoms in patients with inflammatory bowel diseases. *Inflammatory Bowel Diseases*, 20(7), 1194–1197.
5 Schreiner, P. Yilmaz, B., Rossel, J.B., et al. (2019). Vegetarian or gluten-free diets in patients with inflammatory bowel disease are associated with lower psychological well-being and a different gut microbiota, but no beneficial effects on the course of the disease. *United European Gastroenterology Journal*, 7(6), 767–781.
6 Gerbault, P., Liebert, A., Itan, Y., Powell, A., Currat, M., Burger, J., Swallow, D.M. & Thomas, M.G. (2011). Evolution of lactase persistence: an example of human niche construction. *Philosophical Transactions of the Royal Society of London. Series B, Biological Sciences*, 366(1566), 863–877.
7 Regueiro, M., Greer, J.B. & Szigethy, E. (2017). Etiology and treatment of pain and psychosocial issues in patients with inflammatory bowel disease. *Gastroenterology*, 152(2), 430–439.e4.

2 Stress and the Gut

IBDs are biological disorders, so you may be wondering what role, if any, stress has to play. You certainly don't want to be told your symptoms are all in your head. And there are few things more frustrating and upsetting than being told your symptoms are somehow your *fault*. Old, outdated psychoanalytic models often blamed physical symptoms on *neurosis*. Gee, if you just weren't so *neurotic* then your gut wouldn't hurt, right? This is obviously nonsense, and it's the sort of approach that gave psychiatry and psychology such a bad name for so long in the public's mind.

The information outlined is this chapter is very different. It is based on a modern, scientific, biomedical understanding of how the brain and body mount a biological response to perceived threat. We now understand a lot more than we used to about how all the various systems in our bodies (the brain, the gut, the endocrine system and more) are linked to each other and have reciprocal effects on each other that *mostly* serve us quite well, but don't always.

The Enteric Nervous System

Did you know that you have a brain in your gut? Well, not really. But many gastroenterologists point out that the gut has its own nervous system that has just as many nerve cells, or neurons, as the spinal cord! The enteric nervous system consists of a number of different types of neurons that do different jobs. For example, motor neurons are embedded in the muscles in the digestive tract, and control motility – the smooth contractions of muscles that move food through the system at just the right speed (peristalsis) and the mixing, squishing actions that help break food down, mix it up, expose it to digestive juices and make it available for absorption (segmentation contractions). Sensory neurons do lots of different jobs, including sensing or "tasting" different chemicals in the food you have eaten (like glucose and the amino acids that make up proteins), conveying information about stretch and tension in the walls of the stomach and intestines, and also relaying the perception of pain.

Not surprisingly, people with chronic gut ailments become much more sensitive to the sensations that arise in the enteric nervous system. This means several things.

DOI: 10.4324/9781003057635-3

1   People with GI problems are more likely to *notice* even normal activity in the gut. Most people are not aware of peristalsis or segmentation contractions or gas bubbles moving along. But living with an IBD tends to focus the person's attention on their gut, and sometimes even normal sensations may seem to suggest that there's a problem going on, even if there isn't. This is called *visceral hypersensitivity*, because people become hypersensitive to sensations in their viscera, or gut, notice them more frequently and often start to worry about them. Somewhere between 50% and 70% of patients with IBD will have abdominal pain when their disease is actively in flare. Research suggests that even subtle inflammation and, subsequently, pain can be present even when standard disease activity indices suggest that the disease is in remission. Finally, as mentioned in Chapter 1, having an IBD can result in the brain turning up the volume on pain sensations from the gut, a problem that can persist when there is no active inflammation and that overlaps considerably with IBS.

2   Unfortunately, you are more likely to develop visceral hypersensitivity if you have a history of GI disease like Crohn's or colitis. This is partly because paying attention to gut symptoms may have been important in monitoring and tracking your symptom severity and response to medication and other treatments. This *taught* you to pay attention to visceral sensations. But it's also because hypersensitivity of the primary sensory neurons in the gut may actually cause changes in the central nervous system, causing pain neurons to fire more easily. All these nerve systems interact with each other, and have actual biological effects on each other via specific mechanisms like membrane proteins and cytokines. The details are less important than understanding that there really are specific biological processes that can lead people with IBDs to develop hypersensitivity to abdominal sensations and pain.

3   Once you develop visceral hypersensitivity, both the sensory and motor neurons may start to overreact or respond too strongly to certain kinds of foods and to stress. A meal that might leave a person without GI issues feeling slightly overfull might send a person with GI problems rushing to the bathroom as the enteric nervous system reacts with all kinds of loud, mixed up signals registering the overload of fat and rushing the barely digested meal through the system.

4   Once sensory and pain receptors in the gut become overly excitable, these receptors scream, *"ARE YOU TRYING TO KILL ME!?"* after that meal, where the receptors in a person without GI issues might just murmur "enough already." Pain grabs our attention. It's usually a signal that something is really wrong, and that we'd better do something to get ourselves out of harm's way. In fact, pain is a really important way of protecting ourselves. Your hand hurts when you put it on the hot stove, and that instantly triggers a reflex to pull your hand away, sparing you a bad burn. Some people are born without the ability to sense pain (called congenital insensitivity to pain). This sounds like a blessing, but it's really a curse. Many of these people suffer

horrible disabling or disfiguring accidents and very few survive past age 25. So pain can be an important signal and can give us information that something is wrong that has to be fixed. Like a smoke detector, pain tells us there's a fire to put out.

On the other hand, overly sensitive pain receptors are *not* providing any useful information. They are more like smoke detectors that go off every time you take a shower or boil water. At best that's noisy and annoying. But what if you gathered up the family and fled the house every single time it happened? You'd spend an awful lot of time feeling panicked and frantic and not much time cooking dinner! Pain receptors in the gut are supposed to tell us when we have a serious infection, an ulcer or fistula, a small bowel obstruction or have eaten something dangerous. They are *not* supposed to overreact to basically benign foods, and they're certainly not supposed to overreact to environmental and psychological stressors. So the real challenge here is figuring out how to tell the *difference* between visceral hypersensitivity (pain and discomfort that don't actually signal anything dangerous), and pain that signals an actual flare-up or complication that requires medical attention or management.

Stress and the Autonomic Nervous System

This would all be bad enough, but the enteric nervous system doesn't operate in an independent vacuum. It is also in constant communication with the rest of the *autonomic nervous system* (or ANS). The rest of the ANS is actually made up of two different, parallel, sets of nerve systems that have to work together in balance with each other. Both of them directly affect the functioning of the intestinal tract and "talk" back and forth with the enteric nervous system.

One is called the *parasympathetic nervous system.*

The other is called the *sympathetic nervous system.*

It's easiest to think about them in terms of the processes they control. The *parasympathetic* nervous system helps us *rest and digest.* Sounds like a good thing! It's responsible for managing lots of body processes that help us feel calm and at ease. This system is active when our brains tells us that everything's going well, no emergencies need attending to, and we can devote our time and attention to sleeping, eating, digesting, and generally hanging around and feeling relaxed.

The *sympathetic* nervous system, on the other hand, helps us with *fight or flight* responses. It's responsible for managing all the body processes that make us feel keyed up, alert and ready for action. This system is active when our brains tell us that there's something dangerous or threatening in our environment that has to be dealt with either by fighting or by running away.

Sympathetic nervous system activation affects the *whole body*. It leads to increases in heart rate, blood pressure, respiration (breathing faster) and muscle tension. Our brains squirt out adrenaline and cortisol and our livers make lots of glucose (blood sugar) available to our muscles. Sympathetic nervous system activation also leads to dumping waste and urine. In a life-threatening emergency, you can't waste resources carrying around extra weight, and you're not worried about extracting those last few nutrients, so the muscles in the stomach, bladder and colon spasm in order to get rid of the waste. That's why people vomit, "pee their pants" or "soil themselves" when they're very frightened.

Believe it or not, this is a *great* system to have in place if you are trying to escape from a saber-tooth tiger. All that activation focuses your attention sharply on the threat and gives you lots of energy and power to fight (or run!) for your life. Unfortunately, it's not really a very good system to have in place if you're dealing with family conflict, or rush hour traffic, or unpaid bills. That is, most of the "threats" we face in modern life don't require a massive and immediate physical effort to manage. But that doesn't stop your body from reacting to a difficult meeting with your boss, or an argument with a loved one the same way our ancestors' bodies reacted to an encounter with a saber-tooth tiger!

This means that our body's physical response to *stress* isn't always very helpful. We get all juiced up, and then have nowhere to go with all that activation. This is why people who are chronically "stressed" can experience lots of different physical symptoms, like muscle spasms (especially in the neck, shoulders and back), headaches, chest pain, hives, heartburn, indigestion and gut problems. For people with chronic GI issues, the main "symptom" of sympathetic nervous system activation may be acute awareness of the effect on the gut. You *feel* the spasms in your colon. It can feel like you suddenly, urgently need to defecate, and it can be uncomfortable or even painful. These symptoms are *real* and are the direct result of your body's physical response to stress.

Not surprisingly, lots of research in the area of irritable bowel syndrome has shown that *stress* is very closely linked to IBS symptom severity. For folks with an IBD who have developed secondary IBS, this may be equally true for you. Again, this does *not* mean that your symptoms are "all in your head" or that you are just "neurotic." Your IBD may be in remission, but you really are still suffering from physical GI symptoms. Remember, we now understand a lot more about how psychological stress has a *physical* effect on the digestive system, particularly in people with a predisposition to visceral hypersensitivity.

The role of stress in exacerbating the symptoms of IBDs themselves is much less clear. Stress definitely does not *cause* Crohn's or colitis. Someone with an IBD might find that during a particularly stressful time in their life their IBD actually remains in remission and they have few or no symptoms of GI distress. They might also find that during a happy, relatively stress-free period, their IBD suddenly flares out of the blue. On the other hand, there is some evidence that stress in the environment can increase inflammation throughout the body, including the GI system, and might trigger a flare that you wouldn't otherwise have experienced. Moreover, people with IBDs are often already experiencing cramping and diarrhea, and stress can certainly trigger those symptoms in healthy people who don't have an IBD. So it makes sense that stress could potentially *worsen* symptoms in someone with an IBD.

Chronic Inflammation

Another recent advance in our understanding of GI problems is the role of chronic, *low-grade* inflammation and the degree to which stress and stress hormones contribute to the inflammatory process. *Inflammation* is actually the result of processes the body engages in to *protect* itself and heal from tissue damage or infection. In the short term, normal inflammation is quite helpful. Indeed, failure of the body to generate an inflammatory response is linked to some serious diseases and can make us more vulnerable to or can prolong infections. But *chronic inflammation* is clearly not good for us. In chronic inflammation, the inflammatory response is either too strong, goes on too long, or is directed at the wrong targets. Many diseases and conditions in modern society are actually the result of chronic inflammation that is misdirected in some way. Examples include allergies, asthma, rheumatoid arthritis, lupus and multiple sclerosis, as well as the inflammatory bowel diseases.

Recent research suggests that corticotrophin releasing factor (CRF), which is released by the brain when we are stressed, may modulate intestinal inflammation. There are CRF receptors in the brain *and* in the gut itself. CRF receptors may be components of the inflammatory processes in both IBD and IBS. CRF is released in the brain in response to stressors and helps activate the hypothalamic–pituitary–adrenal (HPA) axis, a crucial part of the stress response system. In fact, these structures are important parts of the endocrine system I mentioned earlier. Brain CRF also acts on the autonomic nervous system. In addition, the gut contains CRF sensors that contribute to stress-related exacerbation of GI symptoms in both IBD and IBS. This shared vulnerability may be why IBD patients are more likely than the general population to develop IBS. It also helps explain why symptoms of IBD can include fatigue and joint pain and skin problems, all of which are the result of inflammatory processes throughout the body.

IBD Symptoms as a Stressor

Of course, everyone has to deal with life stress. But when you throw IBD symptoms into the mix, things get even worse. Symptoms like fatigue and joint pain can make you feel less resilient in general, more demoralized and less able to cope with whatever life throws at you. In addition, GI symptoms can make something that might be somewhat stressful (like a long family car trip or an important meeting) *hugely* stressful. That's because it's natural to worry about the possibility that GI symptoms will really interfere with your ability to do things. But here's the thing. Just as the neurons in your intestinal wall may be sending more "problem signals" than they need to be, it may be that you are entertaining more "problem thoughts" than you need to be.

People with gut problems often develop anxiety about the consequences of having GI symptoms. For example, many people worry about feeling embarrassed if they have to excuse themselves to go to the bathroom frequently.

They worry about offending or disgusting people with smelly bowel movements or farts. They worry that they will be seen as unprofessional or incompetent if their gut acts up during the work day. They worry that they will be seen as weird or antisocial or ungrateful if they decline invitations to dinner, or bring their own food to social events or gatherings. They worry about annoying people and calling unwanted attention to themselves if they have to get up during a class, a movie or a worship service. Beyond these social concerns, many people with gut problems truly fear getting "stuck" someplace without ready access to a bathroom. Trains, planes, cars, large malls, stadiums, theaters or parks can all become anxiety provoking. A casual afternoon shopping with friends or catching a ball game begins to feel like a serious gamble.

"Can I make it through?"
"What if I have an attack?"
"What if I can't get to a bathroom quickly enough?"

Many people with gut problems become experts at scoping out potential bathroom locations. Some people even start consulting "bathroom finder" websites before they venture out of the house. Sometimes, just staying home seems like the safest course of action, but then you give up on life experiences that you would otherwise enjoy.

One of the most stressful things some people with GI problems fear is losing control and having a bowel movement in their clothes. The actual incidence of *fecal incontinence* (FI) is hard to pin down, because most people don't sponta-neously report it to their doctor, probably because such a conversation would feel embarrassing. However, one well designed study of fecal incontinence in IBDs found that 22% of patients (some with Crohn's, some with UC) reported varying degrees of incontinence (which could be as mild as a few uncontrolled farts a week or as severe as daily incontinence of liquid and solid stool).[1] They found that incontinence was clearly correlated with disease activity and was strongly related to actual defects in the internal and external anal sphincter muscles. Another review found that about 24% of IBD patients had experi-enced some degree of FI, compared to about 10% of the general population.[2] Amazingly, only about two out of five people with both IBD and FI ever talk to their doctor about it.

Thus, it's very possible that if your IBD has been severe at times, you may have experienced fecal incontinence during a bad flare. Even if you have never actually experienced it, the possibility may make you understandably anxious.

If you are actually experiencing incontinence *currently*, there are some inter-ventions that can help a lot. These include biofeedback training, pelvic floor exercises, electrical stimulation to enhance muscle strength and conditioning and, as a final resort, surgery. There are several different types of biofeedback training. In one kind, small sensors are placed inside the anus. The sensors detect muscle contractions and translate them into bars or lines on a screen that represent successful contraction. This helps people learn to isolate the relevant muscles and exercise them. You can learn to control the external sphincter muscle – to squeeze it tight to prevent stool from leaking out. In another type of biofeedback, a small balloon is inserted into the anus. It is inflated very gradually, a little more each time, to help people learn to contract the relevant muscles and to gain muscular strength and control. It usually takes at least six sessions for biofeedback to be helpful. Obviously, this is a very personal type of therapy, and the trained physiotherapists who do this work are generally very warm, kind professionals who use humor, but are wonderfully respectful and understanding. This kind of treatment is offered at a number of tertiary care specialized GI clinics, especially those associated with major medical centers. If you're interested in pursuing this, it's worth calling around to university affiliated hospitals or big medical centers in your area to find someone who does it.

Another therapy that sometimes helps with fecal incontinence secondary to poor control of the anal sphincter muscles is electrical stimulation of the sacral nerves. The sacral nerves run from your spinal cord to muscles in your pelvis. These nerves both relay sensation and cause contractions of the rectal and anal sphincter muscles. In the standard sacral nerve stimulation (SNS) protocol, a small device that sends electrical impulses to the nerves is implanted. This actually strengthens the sphincter muscles and can result in increased "wait time" and an increase in both resting and maximum pressure that the sphincter muscles can withstand without releasing. This treatment is usually done only after other treatments, like biofeedback, have been tried and haven't worked, but most patients who get to this point achieve considerable relief, meaning they can control and defer defecating. Not surprisingly, quality of life can improve quite a bit as a result.[3]

There are also surgical options for attempting to repair damaged sphincter muscles. These might include transplanting a small piece of thigh muscle to replace a damaged sphincter, or replacing a damaged sphincter with an artificial, pump operated inflatable cuff. Most people with IBDs won't need to consider these options, but if fecal incontinence is truly interfering with your life, they are certainly options to discuss with your care provider.

What we *do* know about fecal incontinence is that lots and lots of patients *don't mention it* to their doctor. So unless your doctor explicitly asks you about it, you may be suffering in silence. Don't be embarrassed to bring this up! Fecal incontinence often has a big impact on quality of life. There really are treatments that can help with it, so don't be shy about telling your doctor and asking for recommendations for treatment.

If you have experienced fecal incontinence in the *past*, you may have been left with a terrible fear that it will happen again, even if your disease is in remission. In people with visceral hypersensitivity, this can become a *self-fulfilling prophecy*. People notice every sensation, every twinge, every muscle spasm in their gut. These sensations make them anxious, as they anticipate the onset of more serious cramps or pain or urgent diarrhea. As soon as they get anxious, sympathetic and enteric nervous system activation starts, causing more roiling and cramping, and increasing the urge to defecate. Now the person may start to worry about getting to a bathroom. They imagine having another episode of fecal incontinence, and this really gets the worry juices flowing! It would be humiliating! *Horrible!* Even *disastrous!* Before you know it, this person is dashing out of the room, desperate to get to the bathroom "in time." This is stressful stuff!

One thing that can make anxiety about flares and urgency easier to manage is knowing that you can legally access a restroom anytime you need to, no matter where you are. Many states actually have *laws* in place guaranteeing access to restrooms in public spaces and businesses/retail establishments for people with certain medical conditions, especially IBDs. (In fact, the first such law was lobbied for and won in Illinois by the mother of a 14-year-old girl with Crohn's who was denied access to a staff bathroom at a retail store, and did, unfortunately, experience fecal incontinence as a result. Official Restroom Access Acts are typically known as Ally's Law in honor of that girl.) The Crohn's and Colitis Foundation provides "I Gotta Go" or "Can't Wait" cards to every member. Many gastroenterologists' offices also have cards that they provide free of charge. These are all sufficient "medical documentation" that you have an urgent, legitimate need to use a rest room wherever you happen to be. If you are in a retail establishment that doesn't normally provide public restrooms (e.g. a bank) or usually only lets paying customers use the restroom (e.g. a restaurant) you can use the card to legitimize your request to use the facilities. Some people have the card, but have never used it because they think it would be embarrassing. It's important to remember that the vast majority of people are truly kind, sympathetic and helpful. If you simply say "I'm so sorry, but I need to use your restroom – it's a medical emergency," almost everyone will smile and show you the way. If they are hesitant, you can produce the card so they know you're not a thief or a crazy person. Just knowing that you have the authority of law and documentation from a national organization or physician behind you can help when you urgently need a restroom.

Summary

It is important to understand that IBDs are caused by a number of different factors, including genetic vulnerability, autoimmune reactivity, disruptions in the microbiome or bacterial ecosystems in the gut, and chronic inflammation, all of which can contribute to the development of secondary visceral hypersensitivity, or amplified pain processing. Psychological distress in response to external life events or to simply living with an IBD can exacerbate the underlying inflammatory process through many intertwined but straightforward biological mechanisms. So really, things are happening at three different levels – biological, psychological and environmental.

But if you think about it, almost everything in our lives happens simultaneously *at all three levels*. Let's say you are supposed to go to your in-laws' house for dinner. You are getting ready to go, and you're thinking about the last time you were there – how your mother-in-law was critical of you and how she and your father-in-law sometimes snipe at each other. You're feeling a little tense. Then you notice a small, crampy twinge in your gut. Could this be a flare-up? Maybe you shouldn't have eaten lunch. Maybe you should try to go to the bathroom before you get in the car. But what if it takes a while? Then you'll be late, and your spouse will be frustrated and annoyed. Maybe you should just suck it up and go. But then what if you REALLY have to go halfway there? Is there a gas station along the way with a restroom that's not too disgusting? Or what if you have to run to the bathroom the instant you arrive? What if you stink up their powder room? You can always say you're sick. But that will just give your mother-in-law more to criticize. By now your gut is cramping in earnest. It hurts, and you know there's no way you can get in the car without going to the bathroom first.

What's going on here? Clearly, there's an *environmental or social stressor.* Obviously, this person's in-laws are a bit difficult to deal with. Anticipating dealing with this stressor is causing apprehension and a bit of anxiety – that's the *psychological distress* part of the equation. But psychological distress translates directly into sympathetic nervous system arousal, which increases the inflammatory stress response, which interacts with the enteric nervous system to cause some sensory overload and abnormal motility in a gut that's prone to inflammation and may not have enough helpful bacteria on board – that's the *biological* piece. This feeds back through *visceral hypersensitivity* to ensure that the person notices the twinges and spasms. But the twinges and spasms now become stressors in and of themselves, triggering a new onslaught of worrisome thoughts, which in turn trigger more arousal and inflammation, which in turn increases the physical discomfort and the urgent need to defecate. Before you know it, this person is having a full-fledged attack and feels truly sick. Their spouse is alternately sympathetic and annoyed. They may cancel the dinner, leading to bad feelings all around. Or the person may go, feeling drained and exhausted, and then only pick at dinner, fearful of bringing on another attack, and further alienating the difficult mother-in-law.

The point is that what people with IBDs are dealing with is the sum of *all of these processes* put together and happening at the same time. It can be like a perfect storm of stressors, worry, experience and fears interacting with a highly vulnerable GI system. No wonder people with IBDs are somewhat more vulnerable to depression and anxiety than healthy people in the community! That's why learning how to manage stress effectively is an important part of your tool kit for coping with Crohn's and colitis and minimizing the impact GI symptoms have on your life.

The good news is that there are ways to intervene quite effectively to reduce the impact of gut symptoms on your life, and to give you considerable relief from this constant GI related distress. This entire program is designed to teach you skills to manage stress effectively, to reduce the impact of stress on your gut, and to reduce the degree to which your life is limited and defined by having to manage your gut symptoms. So let's get started!

Suggested Activities

Complete the self-report questionnaires in Appendices A and B. This will give you a sense of the degree to which your gut symptoms have become real stressors for you.

Notes

1 Papathanasopoulos, et al. (2013). Severity of fecal urgency and incontinence in inflammatory bowel disease: Clinical, manometric and sonographic predictors. *Inflammatory Bowel Disorders*, 19(11), 2450–2456.
2 Gu, P., Kuenzig, M.E., Kaplan, G.G., Pimentel, M. & Rezaie, A. (2018). Fecal incontinence in inflammatory bowel disease: a systematic review and meta-analysis, *Inflammatory Bowel Diseases*, 24(6), 1280–1290.
3 Moya, P. Arroyo, A. Lacueva, J. Candela, F. Soriano-Irigaray, L. Lopez, A. Gomez, M A. Galindo, I. & Calpena, R. (2014). Sacral nerve stimulation in the treatment of severe faecal incontinence: long-term clinical, manometric and quality of life results. *Techniques in Coloproctology*, 18(2), 179–85.

3　Turn It Off or Burn It Off

Relaxation Training and Physical Activity

It's important to remember that stress can make GI symptoms worse for very straightforward biological reasons. All three parts of the autonomic nervous system (sympathetic, parasympathetic and enteric) talk to each other and work in concert with each other. If you are stressed, the parasympathetic system gets quiet, the sympathetic system goes into overdrive, and the enteric system reacts to the signals the sympathetic system is sending it (through chemicals like cortico-tropin releasing factor or CRF). So stress has a direct, *physical* impact on your body and your gut. We have two choices for managing this flood of hormonal and neuroendocrine soup that juices up our bodies and makes us feel tense, stressed and uncomfortable. We can *turn it off* with relaxation exercises and we can *burn it off* with physical exercises.

Turn It Off! – Relaxation Training

It's important to remember that there are skills you can learn that will help you actively cope with both general life stressors, and with the specific stresses and challenges of living with an IBD. The very first step in active coping is learning how to *turn off* the biological stress response by turning on the *parasympathetic* nervous system. The parasympathetic nervous system is the one that allows for *resting and digesting* in peace. It's the opposite of sympathetic activation (*fight or flight*), which is the body's response to stress. So turning on the parasympathetic nervous system is equivalent to turning *off* the sympathetic nervous system. The behavioral exercises that follow are designed to reduce the physical impact of stress on your body and your GI system, and will help with active coping in all kinds of situations. When practiced regularly and used effectively, they can actually reduce the severity of GI symptoms. They can also help you feel more centered, calm and peaceful, and better able to deal with whatever life is throwing at you in the moment. But keep in mind – this program is not like a pill or medicine you take in the short term. This is a training program designed to teach you a set of skills you can use for the rest of your life to manage stress effectively. If you don't practice these, they definitely won't do you any good.

There are three basic types of relaxation exercises:

DOI: 10.4324/9781003057635-4

1   Deep breathing
2   Progressive muscle relaxation
3   Relaxing imagery

Many people find that they gravitate to one or two of them, but don't much care for the other(s). It's important to try all three at least a few times to see if you can get the feel for it, and see if it works for you. My own personal favorite is deep breathing. Done correctly, deep breathing can really take the edge off sympathetic arousal. It can also be done discreetly, anytime and anywhere – on the bus, in a meeting, after lunch, you name it. When you get good at it, just two or three deep breaths, about 30 seconds' total time investment, can lower your heart rate and blood pressure, suppress adrenaline and cortisol (the major stress hormones) and relax the smooth muscles in your colon.

Some people swear by progressive muscle relaxation. They like the structure of thinking about each major muscle group in turn, alternately tensing and relaxing each muscle. They find that the immediate feeling of warmth and release in the muscles is very relaxing and reassuring. It's a very concrete exercise, and you really feel like you're *doing* something to help your body relax.

Other people, especially those high in imaginal ability, love using relaxing imagery to "take them away" from their stress. Imaginal ability is the degree to which you can create mental images that feel real and vivid to you. The more real your imagery feels, the easier it is to get "caught up" in it and the more relaxing it will be. Imagery can work especially well for people who feel like their body has become "the enemy." If you don't trust your body anymore and feel like it betrays you and causes you nothing but pain and aggravation, deep breathing and progressive muscle relaxation may be frustrating and counterproductive, because they focus you on and in your body. If this is true for you, by all means use imagery for a few weeks instead. But as this program starts to work, it might be worth coming back to deep breathing and trying it again.

Whichever type of relaxation exercise ends up being the most useful to you, give them all a try.

Deep Breathing

Deep breathing is probably the single most effective relaxation exercise there is. The autonomic (or "automatic") nervous system has lots of different parts and affects lots of different processes in the body. All of those parts and processes are functioning automatically all the time without any effort or thought on our part. That's a good thing! If we had to *remember* to keep our heart beating or to keep breathing, we'd be in deep trouble if we got distracted! In fact, we can't really exert direct conscious control over any of these processes, *except the breath*. If I asked you to intentionally raise your blood pressure, or to stop the liver from converting stored glycogen into glucose, you would have no idea what muscle to squeeze to make that happen. The one part of the autonomic nervous system that we *can* bring under conscious control is how we breathe. The good news is that how we breathe is actually wired into the system in such a way that changing how we breathe also changes everything else, including heart rate and blood pressure and adrenaline and cortisol and muscle tension and GI system functioning. In fact, deep breathing is so effective at suppressing arousal that CIA operatives are taught how to do it, because it's how you fool a lie detector test!

Unfortunately, the advice to "just take a deep breath" doesn't work very well for most people. That's because there are two very different ways of breathing. One of them – chest breathing (where your shoulders go up and your upper chest expands) – isn't really deep breathing at all, but it's what most people do when you ask them to take a deep breath. Try it – notice what you actually do when you try to "take a deep breath." Does your chest rise? Do your shoulders move up towards your ears? Taking that kind of breath will *not* help you relax. In fact, believe it or not, it will probably make you *more* tense. That's because chest breathing actually tends to *activate* the sympathetic nervous system, and that's *not* what we want!

Instead, try this. Stand up. Put your hand on your stomach with your belly button in the curve between your thumb and pointer finger. Now just contract your tummy muscles so your hand moves inward. You're not pressing in with your hand, but if your hand is resting lightly in the right place, it should move in and out as you contract that muscle. Don't worry about breathing yet. Just find that muscle, and keep contracting it over and over until you feel some muscle "burn" just under your rib cage. (About six or seven times should do it.) Feel it?

Now try to use that muscle to squeeze the air out of your lungs. As you contract the muscle, exhale sharply, as if you were blowing out a candle. Do this two or three times, then take a break for a few breaths, and then try it again till you get the hang of it. (If you start to get dizzy, just stop and breathe normally for about 15 seconds.)

Now instead of pretending to blow out *one* candle, imagine that you have to blow out *all* the candles on my last birthday cake. That's a *lot* of candles (but I'm not going to tell you exactly how many!). To blow out that many candles, you need to do a really long, extended exhale – between six and eight full seconds. Use the muscle to squeeze the air out of your lungs, but instead of exhaling sharply, exhale *slowly* over a count of six to eight. After you finish exhaling, just relax, and *let the air pour back in*. Inhale for about five to six seconds, and then hold your breath for a second or two. Then exhale again really slowly and steadily. Try to do this four times in a row, very slowly. You should be able to count six to eight seconds while you exhale, inhale for five to six seconds, hold for a second, and then exhale again. There's a rhythm to this:

exhale – 2–3 – 4–5 – 6–7 – 8, inhale – 2–3 – 4–5, hold your breath – 2–3,
exhale – 2–3 – 4–5 – 6–7 – 8, inhale – 2–3 – 4–5, hold your breath – 2–3,
exhale – 2–3 – 4–5 – 6–7 – 8, and so on.

Got it? You should find that as you "relax" after exhaling, you just inhale deeply and slowly without having to think about it too much. Imagine the air pouring into your lungs and filling them from the bottom up, almost like filling a pitcher with water. Now try again, and this time, put one hand on your chest, and the other on your belly. You should find that the hand on your belly moves in and out with each exhale/inhale while the hand on your chest doesn't move much at all. This is called *diaphragmatic* or deep belly breathing. Done correctly, diaphragmatic breathing actually *turns on* the parasympathetic nervous system and *turns off* the sympathetic nervous system. If you're doing it deeply and slowly, you should be taking between four and five breaths per minute, you should feel warm and relaxed, and not dizzy at all. If you start to feel dizzy, you're probably breathing too fast. Just hold your breath a little longer after each inhale.

It may feel very awkward and unnatural at first, but I guarantee your body knows how to do it. It's what you naturally do when you're asleep. (Remember *rest and digest*? Sleeping is all about parasympathetic nervous system control.) The trick is to learn how to harness this consciously so that you can control it, and get the good effects anytime you need a little help managing stress. If you're having trouble getting the feel for it, try practicing lying down. This makes it easier for some people.

If you're the kind of person who likes "data," there's a fun way to incorporate simple biofeedback into this by watching your heart rate rise and fall while you breathe. Either use a device that gives you a pulse reading (a Fitbit, smart watch, exercise heart rate monitor or pulse oximeter) or simply put your fingers on a pulse point at your wrist or neck. During the inhale, your heart will speed up a little, and then during the exhale it will *slow down*. That's the effect of the parasympathetic nervous system. As you slow and deepen your breathing, your overall heart rate will go down, but you'll still notice that it beats faster while you inhale and slower while you exhale. If you can notice that, you're doing it right! Weirdly, the ability to maximize heart rate "variability" (the difference between the slow and fast beats) is a sign of both cardiovascular health *and* good emotion regulation skills. It means you can both rise to a challenge (with sympathetic activation) *and* calm yourself down quickly afterwards (with parasympathetic activation).

If you're really having trouble getting the hang of this, it may be easier to find a guided mindful breathing or breathing focused meditation exercise on the internet. There are many free resources out there that you can play on your computer or smart phone. They vary in length (from just a few minutes up to 45 minutes, with most being in the 10–15 minute range). They also vary in lots of other ways. Some include background music, or colorful kaleidoscopic fractals on the screen. Some are very "new-agey" and some are quite straightforward. Sometimes the speaker talks very slowly and in a gentle, quiet way. Some people love this. Others find it quite annoying. Sometimes the speaker talks normally. Some reference Buddhist origins or Yogic traditions. You don't need to be religious or even spiritual to benefit from these exercises. If you are a member of a different faith tradition, you certainly don't have to buy into the specifics of a foreign faith. There is considerable scientific evidence that paced, mindful breathing is a great way to reduce sympathetic nervous system arousal. It has helpful effects on heart rate and the pattern of your heart beats, and on blood pressure and stress hormones. If you're struggling with intentional diaphragmatic breathing, doing a mindful breathing meditation may be just the ticket. Most people end up doing perfect diaphragmatic breathing by the end of such an exercise without even realizing they're doing it! Just try Googling "mindful breathing" or "breathing meditation" and click on a few different options until you find one you like.

Progressive Muscle Relaxation

Progressive muscle relaxation involves systematically tensing and relaxing the major muscle groups of the body. It may sound a little crazy to *tense* your muscles if you're trying to relax, but we're counting on the fact that tensing your muscles for about ten seconds actually leads to muscle *fatigue*. When you stop tensing the muscle, it will not only relax, it will actually get *more* relaxed than it normally is, because the muscle fibers are tired. This should leave the muscle feeling quite lax, but also warm and vital.

Try to tense each major muscle group, in order, for about ten seconds. Pay attention to how the muscles feel when they are tensed, compared to how they feel when you release the tension and let them relax. You should wait at least 10–15 seconds between each muscle group. In general, start with a muscle group on one side of your body, then do the same muscle group on the other side of the body.

1 Sitting in a comfortable chair, hold your right arm out over your lap, make a fist, bend it up toward the ceiling, and tense the lower right arm and wrist muscles as tightly as you can for ten seconds. Then relax your arm and let it drop into your lap. Now do the same thing with your left arm.
2 Bring your right hand up to your shoulder and tense the muscles in your upper arm, as if you were a body builder showing off your biceps. Tense and hold tight for ten seconds, then release. Now do the same thing with your left arm.
3 Hold your right leg out in front of you, point your toes, and tense your calf muscle as tightly as you can. Hold for ten seconds and then release. Then do the same thing with your left leg.
4 Extend your right leg straight out, flex your foot (point your toes towards the ceiling) and tense your thigh muscle as tight as you can for ten seconds, then release. Do the same thing with your left leg.
5 Now put your knees together, squeeze your thighs together, and clench the muscles in your bottom as tight as you can for ten seconds. Then release.
6 Still sitting in your chair, round your back by pulling your abdominal muscles in as tight as you can and press the small of your back into the back of the chair. Hold for ten seconds and then release.

7   Stand up, clasp your hands together behind your back, and pull your hands down and out behind you, pulling your shoulder blades together as far as you can. This should tighten the muscles in your back while simultaneously stretching the muscles in your chest. Hold for ten seconds and release.

8   Now hold your right arm in front of you across your chest so that your right hand juts out past your left shoulder. Grab your right elbow with your left hand, and pull your arm into your chest. Hold for ten seconds and release. Now do the same thing with your left arm, grabbing your left elbow with your right hand.

9   Drop your head down in front and pull your shoulders forward and down. Hold for ten seconds and release.

10 Finally, tense the muscles in your forehead and face by lifting your eyebrows up toward your hairline and opening your eyes as wide as you can. Hold for ten seconds and release.

A nice way to combine imagery and muscle relaxation is to use imagery to help you visualize a warm, relaxing feeling slowly moving up your body from your toes to the very top of your head. Instead of systematically tensing and relaxing your major muscles, you just focus on very small body parts in sequence, feeling them and trying to imagine letting all the tension go from that particular body part. Some people like to visualize a warm, golden light warming each part in turn until your whole body is bathed in relaxing warmth and you feel entirely limp and heavy, like honey in the sun. One of the tricks to this exercise is to try to relax body parts we don't normally think we can really control (like your big toe or your hips or your ears). This helps avoid the pitfall of inadvertently tensing a muscle just because you're focusing on it.

Start with the big toe on your right foot. Then move to the big toe on your left foot. Slowly introduce the rest of the toes, followed by the ball of your foot, the arch of your foot, the heel and the ankle, going back and forth between left and right. Really take a second or two to focus your attention on that particular part of your body. When's the last time you focused on the feelings in your left heel? Let your mind center in that part for a moment, feeling the tension draining out, before you move on to the next body part. Move up your leg, imagining first the shin and then the calf of each leg being bathed in warm, golden light. Imagine your knees relaxing in front and in back. Take your time. Then imagine your thighs relaxing, then your hips, your bottom and the small of your back. Move up your back to your shoulder blades, and up through your shoulders down your arms to your elbows, your forearms, your wrist, your thumbs and each finger in turn. Then come back up to your neck, and imagine the warm light relaxing your chin, and your lips, and your nose and your ears and your eyebrows and your hair. By the time you've made it up to the top of your head, you should feel warm and limp and very languid. Ideally, you'll be doing slow diaphragmatic breathing too, without even having realized that you're doing it!

Relaxing Imagery

Another thing a lot of people find relaxing is to imagine themselves in a place that they find very soothing and peaceful. For some people, the beach is perfect. Other people like to imagine themselves in the woods, or on top of a mountain, or in their grandmother's kitchen, or in a luxurious hotel suite with a private Jacuzzi, or even floating around in a warm, lavender cloud. Whatever you pick, make sure it feels like a safe, peaceful place to *you*. You should also pick something that you can imagine vividly and in detail, using the four senses of sight, hearing, touch and smell. For example, if you're imaging being at the beach, try to see the play of light and shadow on the sand and notice how the color and shapes in the sand change as you walk down toward the water. The sand starts out dry, soft and warm with big, shapeless dimples where people have walked. As you get closer to the water, the sand gets darker, cooler, flatter and slightly harder. When you get all the way down to the water, the sand gets squishy and wet. Listen to the waves crashing or lapping at the sand, and the sound of sea birds calling, and the rustling of the wind in the dune grasses. Smell the clean, tangy, salty smell of the sea. Feel the warm sun on your back, the cool breeze on your cheek, the soft sand underfoot or the water slipping around your toes. Involve yourself in the image. Imagine running along the beach, or scooping up handfuls of water and watching the sunlight shatter into a million diamonds as you throw the water up into the air. The more involved, detailed, and vivid you can make the image, the more relaxing the exercise will be.

A nice way to combine imagery with deep breathing is to imagine the waves rolling in to the beach in time with your breath. Watch each wave as it begins to surge, comes up in a crest, crashes onto the beach, and then gets pulled back out to sea, sucking at the pebbles and licking at the sand. You can imagine inhaling as the wave surges and crests, exhaling as it crashes and flows back out, and then pause for a count or two as the next wave begins to surge.

Burn It Off! – Physical Activity

The other major way to manage the physical effects of stress is with physical activity. Remember that the reason the whole sympathetic nervous system developed (and has been conserved over hundreds of millions of years of vertebrate evolution) is primarily to help us escape predators. Escaping from a predator requires us to *freeze*, to *flee*, or to *fight*. Fleeing and fighting in particular require a massive burst of physical energy. That what that whole neuroendocrine stress soup is there to do! It raises blood pressure and heart rate, increases respiration, floods us with oxygen, glucose, adrenaline and cortisol, and ensures that we can run away from that saber tooth tiger or, if we must, bash it over the head with our mammoth bone club. This is a *great* system to have in place when the major stressors in your life are tigers or stampeding wildebeest. It is *not* a great system to have in place when the major stressors in your life are overdue bills, or bad bosses or teenagers who won't do their homework or their chores. In other words, the stressors of modern human life typically don't require a massive physical effort to survive them.

Unfortunately, we are still stuck with the same vertebrate stress response system as mice and rabbits. That means that the very best way to *burn off* that uncomfortable neuroendocrine soup that leaves us tense and wound up and terribly uncomfortable is to use it for what it was intended for – physical activity!

Now, let's acknowledge that lots of people experience physical exercise as really hard and fairly unpleasant. We all know we *should* exercise, and often feel guilty when we don't, but lots of people just can't get themselves to do it. And exercise is particularly difficult if you've been ill, or if you are still experiencing significant fatigue or joint pain, or if you have frequent diarrhea, or malabsorption issues that lead to anemia or low weight. But gentle, regular physical activity is still going to be one of the best ways to help yourself feel better in the face of life's challenges. So let's take a look at each of the common reasons for not exercising.

1   *Exercise is painful.* This is only true if you push yourself too hard. While it can be a little uncomfortable to start a new activity routine, if you work your way up gently and carefully, physical exercise should never be painful. "No pain no gain" is actually a terrible slogan that leads to injuries and giving up.

2   *Exercise is exhausting.* It is true that expending effort can lead us to feel more tired in the short term, and starting to exercise (literally, putting on your shoes and heading out for a walk) can feel very effortful at the outset. But most people find that gentle physical activity leaves them feeling *more* energized than they would feel if they just spent that time sitting on the couch. And over time, exercise typically gives us *more* energy overall, *and* helps us sleep better.

3   *Exercise is embarrassing.* If you're out of shape, and haven't done much physical activity in a long time, you may not feel very proud of your body, or you may even feel ashamed of how you look or what you can manage to do. You can always start by doing simple physical activities (like stretching, core strengthening, walking up and down the stairs, lifting household weights like soup cans, or doing a yoga video) in the privacy of your own home, or simply go for a walk around the neighborhood.

4   *"I hate going to the gym."* I don't blame you. So do I. I hate staring at myself in all the mirrors (who thought *that* was a good idea!?) I don't love being around dozens of other sweaty people. I dislike the noise of multiple televisions playing. And I hate climbing a stairway to nowhere. So I never go to the gym. I run or walk (in the woods when possible) or bike outside, or use a rowing machine or stationary bike or do yoga in the privacy of my family room.

5   *"I hated sports/I was bad at sports."* So don't play sports! I have never understood the emphasis on organized team sports in gym classes in school. Lots of kids grow up hating "gym class" because they got picked last for

the team, or couldn't pass or dribble or hit the ball. Almost no one continues doing any of those activities once they leave secondary school. It would make much more sense to focus on lifetime health and fitness activities, including walking, biking, yoga and Pilates, and maybe running and tennis and swimming – things people can actually do on a regular basis as they become adults.

6   *"I loved sports when I was a kid but I can't do them now."* So don't play sports! For those of you out there who *were* athletes, you may miss the competence and camaraderie, or even the competitive thrill of team sports. While there are adult leagues for softball, soccer and basketball, if you haven't played in years you're probably better off starting slow and gentle with individual activities like biking or jogging.

7   *Exercise is demoralizing.* "I'm in such terrible shape." "I can barely do anything." "Why even bother?" It is true that starting a habit of regular physical activity takes a bit of self-discipline at the beginning, and doesn't really start to pay off for a few weeks. Like most good things in life, you have to invest a bit of effort up front before you start to get the rewards down the road. But if you stick with it, you *will* see improvement, and you will actually start to look forward to your long walks, or your stretching sessions.

8   *"I guess I'm just lazy."* I hear this from people all the time, and I always tell them that "lazy" is just not a good explanation. First, it's a character flaw, and there isn't really anything to be done about it. Second, it doesn't really explain anything and it doesn't give us any idea how to help motivate you. Motivation is really the result of what we believe the impact of doing and not doing the behavior will be. Most of the thoughts people have about exercise (see above!) are that it will be more punishing than it is rewarding. If you're thinking "Well, I could go to the gym, but it will feel awful and be embarrassing and I'll be exhausted and feel sick afterwards and really what's the point?" then why on earth would you do it? That has nothing to do with being *lazy* and everything to do with how you're thinking about it. If instead, you thought to yourself, "If I go for a 20-minute walk I will really enjoy the fresh air. It would be easier to sit here on the couch, but if I go my back will feel better and I'll actually feel less stressed and a bit more energized and less like a lump." That seems much more appealing, doesn't it? Wouldn't you be more likely to "exercise" if you thought about it that way?

All of these negative thoughts about exercise can be countered with more realistic, more helpful thoughts. Physical activity should never be exhausting or painful. It need not be embarrassing or demoralizing. Gentle physical activity – even just going for a walk or doing some easy stretching in your home before bed – can go a long way toward reducing the impact of chronic stress and inflammation on your body and your mind.

Summary

In Chapter 2 we mapped out the biological reasons that stress can exacerbate physical symptoms and discomfort in the gut. Because of the powerful neurological connections between the brain and the gut, stress management is an important part of treatment for IBDs. One important part of stress management is behavioral – relaxation exercises and physical activity that actually reduce the biological impact of chronic stress on our bodies by *turning it off* and *burning it off*. There are three basic types of relaxation exercises you can learn that will help you turn stress off.

1   Deep breathing
2   Muscle relaxation
3   Imagery

Most people find that they gravitate most naturally to one or another. Some people love deep breathing. They find it easy to learn, they can do it unobtrusively, and it quickly reduces stress and the physical arousal and discomfort associated with stress. On the other hand, trying to focus on breathing is boring or confusing for some people. They just can't seem to get the knack of it, at least not when they're trying to do it consciously. Some people love muscle relaxation. Other people find that it just focuses their attention on all their aches and pains and even heightens visceral sensitivity. If you feel like your body has become your enemy, and betrays you at every turn, then focus on imagery, at least at the beginning. Most people find that they prefer one over the other two, or that a combination of two works great, but they hate the third one. The point is that you need to experiment until you find the package that works well for *you*.

Relaxation is a learned skill, like learning to ride a bicycle. With regular practice you become better at it and will be able to *turn stress off*. If you cannot, or will not, practice regularly, then you probably won't get much benefit from it. Once you learn this skill, however (and it usually just takes a few weeks to get good at it), it's something you'll have available to use to help you manage and reduce the physical impact of stress for the rest of your life! Even a 30-second "time out" during a stressful day to take two or three deep breaths and imagine yourself on the beach can do wonders for reducing or even turning off your body's response to stress.

Physical activity is the other half of reducing the biological effects of stress. By *using* all that activation and arousal for exactly what it evolved for, you can *burn stress off*. Physical activity doesn't have to be intense to work. In fact, gentle, low impact activities like walking can be quite effective at reducing stress. If you're curious, and want to try something new, yoga can particularly helpful as well. But the main idea is to find something you like, do it regularly, and stick with it. Bike through a beautiful park. Go for a walk with a friend. There are lots of possibilities. Don't let your IBD steal your body from you. Reclaim it.

Suggested Activities

Practice deep breathing, progressive muscle relaxation and imagery at least once a day, every day for a week, for at least five to ten minutes. Lots of people like to do it shortly before bedtime, since it's very soothing, and often helps people fall asleep. In fact, some people initially find it easier to practice deep breathing when they're lying down.

Pick a physical activity you can try and do it at least *once* this week. It could be as simple as going for a walk. Pay attention to how you feel before and afterwards. If it feels good, try it again. If you didn't love it, think about what else you could try.

In addition to practicing the techniques, keep some notes about how it's going. Over the week, take a few moments to enter in the box on the next page a bit about how the relaxation exercises and physical activity are going for you. Taking the time to write about your experiences can help you think about what you've learned and can point you in the right direction as you continue developing these skills.

My experiences with relaxation exercises and physical activity

---

In the next chapter, we'll start exploring the kinds of situations that tend to be stressful for you. The way you respond to these situations will be explored and alternative responses and reactions that minimize stress will be discussed.

4   The Cognitive Model of Stress Management

You should continue practicing relaxation exercises at least three to four days a week for the rest of the program. Feel free to use only the components that work well for you. You should also try to gently increase the physical activity you engage in. Shoot for 20 minutes of focused activity at least three to four days a week.

Cognitive Model of Stress

Behavioral management of stress (through things like relaxation and physical activity) is great, but it will only get you so far. Relaxation can only reduce the physical impact of stress you're already experiencing, and physical activity can only reduce the impact of arousal on your body. Wouldn't it be better to reduce the actual stress itself?

You may have tried to do this by curtailing certain activities (like traveling, shopping or going to shows) or avoiding certain situations (like restaurants, parties or other social gatherings, especially if they involve food). The problem with this strategy is that you end up missing out on *life*. Really living means being involved in life, not avoiding it. So rather than reducing stress by trying to *avoid* stressful situations, I'd like to teach you a better way to reduce stress by making potentially distressing situations less stressful to begin with!

Try the following exercise:

Imagine that you are walking down the street, and you see a casual friend walking on the other side of the street, going in the opposite direction. You wave. Your friend does not wave back. Try your best to visualize such a scene as vividly as possible.

How do you react? Take a moment to think about this, and try to identify what would go through your mind and what kind of emotions you might experience if you found yourself in this situation. Enter your reactions into the text box below.

How would I react if I found myself in this situation?

DOI: 10.4324/9781003057635-5

Interestingly, different people might have lots of different reactions in this situation. Some people might be angry. Some people might be sad. Some people might feel anxious. Some people might feel faintly amused. Some people might feel nothing at all. How can different people respond so incredibly differently to what appears to be the exact same situation?

The key, of course, is that it depends on what the person is *thinking* about the situation. If you think to yourself, "Look at that arrogant jerk. I can't believe he would just ignore me that way!" you are likely to feel angry. If, on the other hand, you think to yourself, "Wow – she must really not like me. Something must be wrong with me. I'm uninteresting, unattractive, geeky – I suck..." you are likely to feel sad or even depressed. If you think to yourself, "Oh my gosh! I must have really screwed up to make her angry with me. I wonder what I did wrong? How am I going to face her this weekend?" you are likely to feel anxious. On the other hand, if you think to yourself, "I guess she didn't see me. Oh well, I'll say hi to her next time I see her," then you're not likely to feel much of anything. But if you add in the thought, "Gosh, I wonder if other people saw me waving at 'nobody' and think I'm crazy?" then you might feel embarrassed.

The point is that it is not really the objective situation *itself* that determines how we feel. All the people above experienced exactly the same objective reality. They waved, and their friend did not wave back. Their emotional response was determined by their *beliefs* about the situation. These thoughts, also known as *cognitions*, are very powerful. They cause us to feel emotions and even act in certain ways based on our beliefs about events. If you think the person is being deliberately mean and ignoring you, you may feel angry, and you may act coldly toward the person next time you see them. If you think that there is something wrong with you, or that you screwed up somehow, you may feel sad or anxious, and you may cry or try to avoid the person. The key thing to understand is the connection between the objective situation, your beliefs, and your feelings.

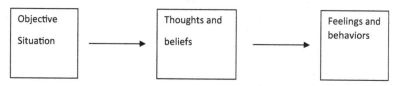

Figure 4.1

Now try to apply this to a real situation from your own life.

Think about a recent situation or event that was stressful for you – something recent enough that you can remember it reasonably well. This may or may not also be a situation in which your gut acted up. Try to describe the situation as objectively as possible in the text box below.

Describe a recent situation that you experienced as stressful:

Now try to identify what you *thought* in response to the situation. Examples include any *beliefs* you had about the situation – like about why it happened or how it was likely to end, any *judgments* you made about yourself or others (e.g. "I really screwed up" or "I should or shouldn't have…" or "She said that on purpose to hurt me") or any *predictions* you might have made (e.g. "I bet I failed the exam" or "He must think I'm really stupid") and so on. Write down these thoughts in the box below.

What thoughts did you have in response to the situation?

Now try to identify all the different emotions you felt. Be careful here! In English, it's perfectly grammatical to say, "I feel like I failed the exam," but that's a thought – not a feeling. You are *thinking* that you might have failed the exam – so that belongs in the thoughts box, not the emotion box. That thought may make you *feel* sad and anxious. Sadness and anxiety are *emotions* and they go in the feelings box. Some people have a lot of difficulty identifying their emotions. Here's a cheat sheet of emotion words to help you out. (We're focusing on negative or unpleasant emotions here, since we're mostly worried about stressful experiences. Of course, there are lots of positive emotions too.)

Sadness	*Fear*	*Anger*
Unhappy	Apprehensive	Annoyed
Upset	Worried	Frustrated
Sad	Anxious	Irritated
Discouraged	Nervous	Aggravated
Miserable	Scared	Angry
Depressed	Terrified	Furious
Hopeless	Petrified	Enraged

Now thinking about the situation you identified, and the thoughts you had, fill in the feelings you experienced in the text box below. You can certainly use words that aren't on the cheat sheet if they seem to capture your feelings better, just be sure you're describing emotions, not thoughts! If the situation also seemed to lead to an increase in your gut symptoms, note that in this box too.

What feelings did you have in response to the situation?

Ideally, you should be able to see the connection between your thoughts and your feelings. In fact, every feeling in the feelings box should be tied to at least one thought in the thoughts box. If there are feelings you identified that don't seem to be tied to a thought, it probably means you haven't really identified all the thoughts you had. For example, imagine that a person has just taken an important exam or test of some kind. They might do the following analysis of what happened.

Situation	Thoughts	Feelings
Took exam	I think I did badly	Anxious Disappointed Hopeless Guilty

If you try to connect each of the feelings to a thought, here's what happens.

Situation	Thoughts	Feelings
Took exam	I think I did badly ⟶	Anxious Disappointed Hopeless Guilty

It may be obvious why the person feels anxious and disappointed. But why does the person feel hopeless and guilty? To understand where those feelings are coming from, the person has to dig a little deeper into what they were thinking.

Situation	Thoughts	Feelings
Took exam	I think I did badly. ⟶ This means I won't get what I want professionally ⟶ I screwed up by not ⟶ preparing more	Anxious Disappointed Hopeless Guilty

When the analysis is complete, you should be able to draw an arrow from a thought to a feeling for every feeling you experienced. Try this now with the situation from your own life that you wrote about above. Be sure that each of the feelings you experienced is "explained" by a thought.

Situation	Thoughts	Feelings

The interesting thing about feelings is that they are not right or wrong. They just *are*. That is, they are the inevitable consequences of our beliefs and thoughts. Beliefs, however, *can* be right or wrong.

Just because we believe something doesn't make it true even if we believe it very strongly and feel very certain that we are right.

Think back to the hypothetical situation we presented at the beginning of the chapter. A person might be thinking all kinds of negative, upsetting things about why their friend didn't wave. They may be absolutely convinced that the friend ignored them on purpose and they may be very upset as a result. If in fact the friend just didn't see them, then the person will be upset *for no reason*. That is, they will be experiencing a whole lot of unnecessary stress. There is an objective reality out there. Either their friend saw them or they didn't. How can you tell? In the heat of the moment, it can sometimes be difficult or even impossible to know. That's why we usually just accept our first gut response, or *automatic thought*, without really examining or questioning it.

The key to reducing unnecessary stress in your life is to make sure that your beliefs are as accurate as possible. All of us "jump to conclusions" sometimes. If you can catch yourself, and try to see situations in alternative ways, you may save yourself a lot of pain. The problem is, we usually don't think about *benign alternatives*, or other ways of looking at the situation that are less upsetting, once we've started to have an emotional reaction. If you're already angry and sad because you think you're being ignored, it may not occur to you that maybe the person didn't see you. The instant you have a negative thought, it may start a cascade of reactions, including both negative emotions and physical symptoms. This makes it hard to think objectively and clearly in the heat of the moment. An important way to practice this is to think about the situation later and see if other, less stressful ways of thinking about it occur to you. For example, our hypothetical person might have done the following analysis:

Situation	Thoughts	Feelings	Benign alternatives
Friend did not wave to me on street	She's ignoring me	Embarrassed	Maybe she just didn't see me
	She must not like me that much	Sad	
	Maybe she doesn't think I'm "cool" enough to be friends with	Frustrated	
	People are so judgmental and cruel	Angry	

Now try to do a similar analysis with the situation you described from your own life. See if you can come up with *benign alternatives* to the *automatic thoughts* you identified. Try to list at least one benign alternative in the box below.

Situation	Thoughts	Feelings	Benign alternatives

People run into several different problems when they start learning to do this.

Occasionally people just can't think of any other way to interpret or understand the situation than their initial take on it. There are several ways to solve this. First, imagine that a friend came to you with a similar situation. What would you say to them? Often it is easier to see alternatives for other people than it is for ourselves. Another way to solve this is to run it by an actual friend or partner, and see if they have another take on it. Try not to bias them by telling them off the bat what *you* thought. Just describe the situation as objectively as possible, and ask them what they think might have been going on. Even if they don't come up with a *benign* alternative, they may come up with a *different* set of thoughts than you had. The very fact that there is at least one alternative way of looking at the situation may help you come up with others.

One strategy that usually doesn't work very well is just to say the opposite of the original thought. For example, if your boss was short with you in the hallway and didn't smile, you might be thinking that he or she is angry with you or dissatisfied with your work. That thought is pretty anxiety provoking, and will probably stress you out. It's not very powerful to just say, "Well, maybe he's not angry with me." This is just contradicting the worrisome thought. It's not really providing an *alternative explanation* for your boss's behavior, so it's not very reassuring. It would be much more powerful to remind yourself, "Oh right, she's got a big presentation to make to the VP tomorrow – maybe she's just stressed about that," or, if you don't *know* of anything that might explain it, to remind yourself that there may be many other alternatives like, "Maybe there's something going on in his personal life or maybe he just got reamed by someone else. It could have nothing to do with me." Most of us have been short with someone at some point because we were stressed out about something that had nothing to do with them. This is more believable than the simple, "Maybe she's not angry at me," because it doesn't ignore the actual objective behavior – your boss did not smile or engage you in conversation. It takes the objective behavior into account, but then provides a more benign *explanation* of why it happened and what it meant.

Another problem that people run into is that they can think of benign alternatives, but they just don't *believe* them. "Sure, I suppose it's possible that s/he just didn't see me, but I don't really think so." Something about the situation convinces you that the more stressful interpretation is the correct one. You may be right. How can you tell? *Examine the evidence.* In the waving friend situation, you might think back to the last contact you had with the person. If s/he called you two days ago to set up a get together over the weekend, it's unlikely that s/he's deliberately ignoring you. If, on the other hand, you've left two voicemails and a text message that haven't been returned, s/he may be trying to tell you something. Sometimes we have screwed up. Sometimes other people have. It may be that it's appropriate to feel distressed about the situation. The question then becomes what to do to fix the problem. Here again, you will find that you have thoughts and beliefs that make you feel more or less optimistic and inclined to take action. Thoughts like "it won't work" or "s/he'll never listen" or "there's no point" or "I can't do it" are likely to undermine your efforts to resolve a problem. The basic lesson here is that, once again, it is your beliefs that matter most in shaping your emotional response and your behavior.

One final type of difficulty people sometimes have with this sort of exercise is that they can think of an alternative, it makes sense, they may even believe it "intellectually," but at the "gut level" they still feel awful. You still feel distressed about the situation and can't shake it. This is usually a clue that there are some other thoughts you haven't identified yet. For example, you might believe that that particular friend really didn't see you on that particular occasion. But what you're really thinking about is how few friends you have, how isolated you feel, and how lonely you'll be this weekend – again. If that's the underlying thought, then convincing yourself that *that* individual didn't see you from across the street won't make you feel any better, because your encounter with that individual is not really why you're feeling so anxious and depressed.

Sometimes when people first hear about these techniques, they think it's a question of learning how to see the glass as "half full" instead of seeing it as "half empty." In fact, cognitive interventions are asking you to do something entirely different. We are asking you to look at the glass and say to yourself:

"It's a 12-ounce glass with six ounces of water in it."

This response is completely, objectively *true*. Both of the traditional responses to this problem are *biased*. One is biased negatively (the glass is half empty) and the other is biased positively (the glass is half full). But the most objective way of looking at it involves no bias at all. How you *feel* about the glass with six ounces of water in it should depend on how thirsty you are! If all you need to do is swallow a vitamin, six ounces of water is more than enough and it's all good. If you just finished an intense workout and are very thirsty, six ounces of water won't be nearly enough. Now you have a concrete problem to solve – you need to get some more water!

That is to say, cognitive interventions are *not* about "pretending" that things are going well even if they're not. In fact, this wouldn't help even if you tried it, because you wouldn't believe it. Rather, cognitive interventions are about helping you learn to see the world as *accurately* and *objectively* as possible. The problem is that many, many people have negative biases or filters that they use to interpret situations in their lives. If you do this routinely and without realizing it, you will be a lot more stressed than you need to be. If you have been entertaining lots of negatively biased automatic thoughts, then seeing the world more accurately should bring about a great deal of relief. In other words:

Don't believe everything you think.

Another nice metaphor for understanding this approach is the following. Imagine that there is a bright yellow lemon sitting on the table in front of you. Now imagine that you have put on a pair of sunglasses with dark blue lenses. What color is the lemon? If you remember your basic art classes from elementary school, you'll remember that yellow + blue = green, and you'll say that the lemon is green. But here's the thing. *Is* the lemon green? Just because the lemon *looks* green to you doesn't mean it has turned green in the real world. The lemon is, of course, still yellow. If you slice into it and taste it, it will still be a lemon, not a bitter green lime. Now imagine that you take off the dark blue glasses and put on lovely rose-colored glasses. Of course, red + yellow = orange. But by now, you know that just because the lemon *looks* orange to you doesn't mean it *is* orange. It's still yellow. If you slice into it now, it will still be a sour lemon, not a nice sweet orange. Negatively biased thinking is like those dark blue sunglasses. It makes things *appear* worse than they actually are. On the other hand, falsely optimistic thinking is like rose colored glasses. It makes things appear better than they actually are. I don't want you to do either one. I want you to see the world the way it actually *is*.

Occasionally people have a very difficult time even understanding why an event or a future possibility has upset them so much. Again, they may be able to identify perfectly sensible, benign alternative ways to think about it, but the deep, gut level distress doesn't seem to abate. Again, this is a clue that you haven't really identified the truly distressing thought. One interesting question to ask yourself in cases like this is, "What's the worst part about this?" or "What would be so terrible about that?" Often, there's some other, deeper belief that is what is really distressing you. For example, you may believe, in your heart of hearts, that it is totally unacceptable to screw up. If you're the guilty party, it may say something terrible about you. If the other person is the guilty party, it may signal betrayal and probably means the permanent end of a friendship. This deeper belief – "It is totally unacceptable to screw up" – should now become the target of your analysis. Is there a benign alternative? There better be, since human beings are not perfect, and screwing up occasionally is inevitable!

Although people do encounter the above difficulties with this sort of exercise, sometimes just putting the thought down in black and white is enough to help you gain a bit more objectivity. A common experience of people doing this sort of exercise for the first time is that the minute they say an automatic thought aloud, or write it down (or hear me echo it back to them), it starts to look and sound exaggerated and even silly. You can recognize immediately that the thought doesn't really make sense. It just doesn't bear up under scrutiny, so you reject it and start to feel better. It's a common experience for patients in my office to look at an automatic thought that we've written on the whiteboard and say, "Well, that's dumb... now that I see it in writing, it just seems goofy." Or I will simply echo a thought back to them and they will say, "Well, when I hear *you* say it, it sounds ridiculous." That's the beauty of this. Since those thoughts usually go totally unexamined and unquestioned, the simple act of identifying and questioning them is sometimes enough to make us feel significantly better.

One final thing to note is that it's very common for people to notice "themes" in their thoughts and feelings. For example, you might notice that you often respond to very different situations with the same basic feeling – maybe anger or anxiety. You may also find that you tend to have very similar thoughts across a range of situations. For example, take three different "stressors" that lots of people might experience – a bad haircut, a mediocre review at work, and a spouse, partner or roommate leaving dirty dishes in the sink. Here are two different sample thought records from two different people.

Amanda

Situations	Thoughts	Feelings	Benign alternatives
Bad hair cut	I look like an idiot. I can't believe how ugly I feel. I'm so unattractive, I never look good no matter how much money I spend	Sad Worthless Anxious	Maybe I didn't explain what I wanted very well. I just expected him to figure it out. Next time, I'll explain what I want more clearly. If I get another bad cut, I'll just find another hairdresser
Mediocre review	I'm just incompetent. My boss thinks I'm an idiot. I never seem to do really well no matter how hard I try	Sad Worthless Anxious	We're *all* really overworked right now because of all the layoffs. I'm trying to do the work of 2½ people here! No wonder I can't get it all done. Maybe my boss and I need to sit down and have a meeting about reasonable expectations
Dirty dishes	I'm such a sucker. Why do I always end up doing the dishes? I must have "doormat" written on my forehead	Sad Worthless Anxious	Maybe I haven't really communicated clearly about how important this is to me

Roger

Situations	Thoughts	Feelings	Benign alternatives
Bad hair cut	That barber is an idiot. I can't believe what a bad job he did. Was he paying any attention at all? I shouldn't even have paid him	Angry Frustrated	Maybe I didn't explain what I wanted very well. I just expected him to remember from last time. Next time, I'll explain what I want more clearly
Mediocre review	My boss is an idiot. I'm working overtime on stuff I wasn't even hired to do, she's too lazy to get me the reports in time to do a good job, and she has the gall to give *me* a bad review!	Angry Frustrated	We're *all* really over-worked and stressed right now because of all the layoffs, including my boss. Maybe she and I need to sit down and have a meeting about reasonable expectations
Dirty dishes	Argh! I can't believe they left the dishes again. That is so incredibly inconsiderate and lazy. I bet they're doing this on purpose just to piss me off	Angry Frustrated	Maybe I haven't really communicated clearly about how important this is to me

You'll notice that Amanda tends to blame herself when things go wrong. She sees *herself* as "an idiot" or "incompetent" or "a sucker." As a result, Amanda often feels sad, worthless and a bit anxious. She also seems to have some difficulty with assertiveness, and she may well be scared of conflict. All of her rational responses suggest that she needs to communicate with people more clearly and assertively. This may make her anxious (she's likely to assume she won't do it well and it won't help) but trying a different strategy is likely to be quite helpful to her across a range of stressful situations in her life.

Roger, on the other hand, tends to blame other people when things go wrong. He tends to think *other* people are incompetent, inconsiderate or lazy. As a result, Roger is often angry and frustrated. Ironically, however, he also seems to have difficulty with appropriately assertive communication. In all likelihood, Roger spends a lot of time fuming quietly, and then occasionally blows up at people when it gets to be too much.

The thing to note here is not only that Amanda and Roger reacted to the same three situations very differently from each other, but that each of them had almost the same reaction *across* the three situations. Amanda ended up feeling sad and worthless, while Roger ended up feeling angry and frustrated across all three situations. Nevertheless, *both* Amanda and Roger could benefit from doing this kind of analysis, and both of them could probably also benefit from communicating more clearly with the people around them and attempting to resolve conflict assertively and appropriately.

You may be wondering what any of this has to do with managing gut problems. Remember that *stress* has a direct effect on the ability of the gut to do its job smoothly and effectively. You can see that both Roger and Amanda are pretty stressed out a lot of the time, although in different ways and for different reasons. It's easy to imagine these situations triggering GI symptoms in both of them. Learning to think about situations more objectively and to consider the benign alternatives can help you reduce the amount of stress you experience in response to life events. Reducing your stress load will make your GI symptoms easier to cope with. I promise.

Suggested Activities

This week you should try to complete three of these "thought records" about three different situations. We call them thought records, rather than situation or feeling records, because we want to emphasize that identifying and questioning your thoughts is the key to reducing unnecessary stress in your life. You can pick any situation that left you feeling the least bit stressed. It could be something relatively trivial (like a bad haircut or someone tailgating you) or something more significant (a difficult meeting at work or a fight with a loved one). Try to describe the situation as objectively as possible, without making any assumptions about other people's motivations or thoughts, causes or outcomes. Next, try to identify all the relevant thoughts you had in response to the situation. Try to identify all the emotions or feelings you experienced in the aftermath. Hopefully, each of the emotions will be tied to and explained by a thought. Finally, try to come up with some alternative explanations or ways of thinking about the situation that might make you feel better.

When you've completed three thought records, read through them one after the other to look for themes in your emotional responses and your thoughts. You may or may not find any. But if you do, it's a big clue that there's something consistent about the way in which you're thinking about things that might be worth changing.

Thought Record

Situation	Thoughts	Feelings	Alternatives and evidence

Thought Record

Situation	Thoughts	Feelings	Alternatives and evidence

Thought Record

Situation	Thoughts	Feelings	Alternatives and evidence

5 Applying the Cognitive Model to GI Symptoms

In the last chapter we focused on how cognitions – what we think and believe about events – can magnify stress and make us feel more upset than necessary. Hopefully, you took the time over the week to write about a few situations in which you were able to identify your thoughts and understand how the feelings you experienced arose directly from your thoughts. You may even have been able to come up with some *alternative* ways of thinking, and to examine the *evidence* for each set of thoughts to determine which was most likely to be true. This week, we are going to see how some of those general skills can be applied directly to the experience of GI symptoms.

One way cognitive interventions can help with gut problems is by reducing your stress burden generally. As you've learned, the lower your general stress level, the less your GI system will be affected by the biological effects of stress and the fewer physical symptoms you should experience. But one of the unfortunate things that happens with gut problems is that GI symptoms are not only a *reaction* to stress, they are also a potential stressor *in themselves*. As with any other experience, we have beliefs and thoughts in response to the situation that can either minimize or magnify how stressful the GI symptoms themselves will be.

People have two different types of thoughts about their GI symptoms.

1   Thoughts about the physical discomfort and symptoms themselves. Examples include things like:

"I can't stand this anymore."
"I'm helpless – there's nothing I can do."
"This is intolerable."
"It's terrible and it's never going to get any better."
"It's not fair."
"If this keeps up I'll go crazy."
"My IBD must be getting worse… I'm going to be really sick."
"My treatments aren't working… this is a disaster."

2   Thoughts about the social and occupational implications of having GI symptoms. Examples include things like:

DOI: 10.4324/9781003057635-6

"I won't be able to go out."

"Even if I do go out, I won't enjoy myself."

"I won't be able to eat or drink."

"I'll make a fool of myself."

"Everyone will think there's something wrong with me."

"I'll be embarrassed or humiliated if I have to leave."

"I'll be mortified if I soil myself."

"No one will understand."

"People will reject me."

"I'll be fired."

"People will think I'm disgusting."

"People will think I'm weak."

"People will think I'm pathetic."

"People will think I'm crazy."

Many of these thoughts lead to intense feelings of *shame* and make people with GI problems very motivated to keep their difficulties *secret* from people around them. Gut problems just seem more disgusting, embarrassing and humiliating than other kinds of problems – like chronic back pain or migraine headaches. As disabling as those conditions might be, they seem "cleaner" somehow and it might seem like it would be easier to let co-workers, friends and others know what was actually up. Unfortunately, shame and secrecy around GI problems can *compound* the stress you experience enormously. If you don't feel you can explain to people around you *why* you need to stop more frequently on road trips, or limit what/where you eat or step out of the classroom or meeting or theater, it can make things that much more difficult. Many people with gut problems make up "excuses" frequently but also worry a lot about the possible social and work-related implications of dealing with their gut issues. These beliefs – that others would be disgusted, that you will be humiliated, that you have to *hide* what's really going on at all costs – are incredibly stressful. We'll address some of these thoughts and beliefs specifically in Chapter 6. For now, you should ask yourself whether you hold these beliefs and in what ways and under what circumstances they may affect you and even limit what you do.

One way to think about all these negative thoughts about GI symptoms is that it sets up a *cycle* in which GI sensations lead to negative automatic thoughts, which lead to increased distress, which leads to a physical stress reaction, which can sometimes increase GI symptoms and always increase stress and make it harder to cope. This is also known as a *vicious circle* (Figure 5.1).

It's a *circle* because you end up back where you started – with increasing GI symptoms and distress. It's a *vicious* circle because every time you loop around, it gets worse, and there's no obvious way out.

The good news is that you already know two places where you can intervene and stop the cycle. One place to cut the circular chain of events is here (Figure 5.2).

You do this with the relaxation exercises you learned in Chapter 3. Relaxation exercises are all about reducing sympathetic nervous system arousal. Since stress leads to arousal, and arousal increases GI distress, then reducing arousal using relaxation

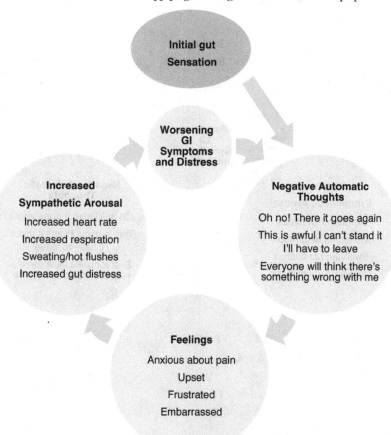

Figure 5.1

techniques should help reduce the impact of stress on your GI symptoms and help you feel more centered and able to cope with whatever is going on.

But remember, an even better way to reduce the impact of stress is to reduce the stress itself! The best way to do this is to target the negative thoughts that are making you feel stressed to begin with. That means you can intervene much earlier in the cycle (Figure 5.3).

You can do this by using the exact same techniques you learned in Chapter 4. In this case, however, the "situation" is always going to include that you have noticed your gut starting to act up or have experienced some other IBD related symptom, sensation or problem. The situation should include some information about the context (e.g. dinner with friends, an important meeting at work, a blind date, results from a lab test). First, you have to identify your own negative thoughts – what went through your mind when you realized your gut was starting to act up? Try this exercise now. Identify a recent episode of GI symptoms and try

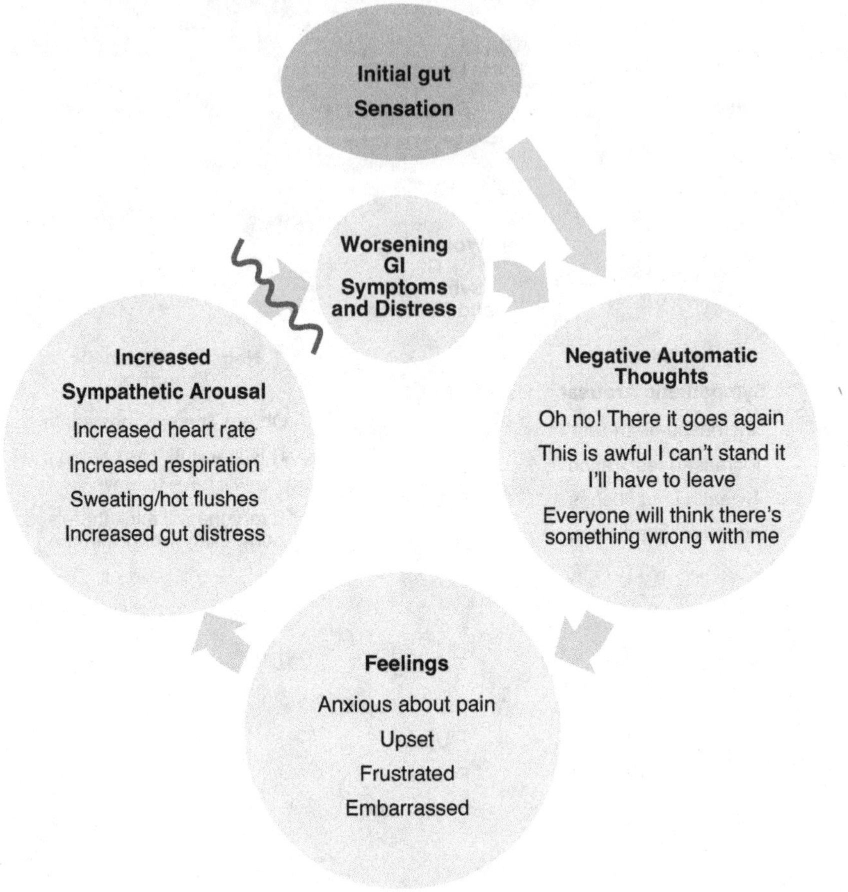

Figure 5.2

to remember what was going through your mind when you first noticed the symptoms. Fill in your negative automatic thoughts and the way they made you feel below:

Situation (including GI symptoms)	Thoughts	Feelings

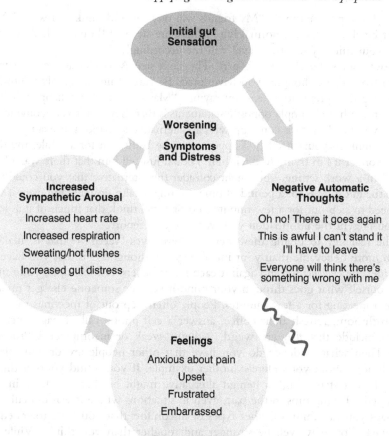

Figure 5.3

It's not always easy to identify our real thoughts and beliefs – especially regarding the things we are anxious or depressed about. You may be having difficulty filling in the "thoughts" part of the worksheet. One useful technique to use here is the "worst case scenario" question. Given the situation you were in, what is the worst possible outcome that you could anticipate or imagine happening? Many people are tempted to give what they think is the "right" answer to this question – something like, "Well, nothing would really happen. It wouldn't be a big deal." If you really believed that, then you probably wouldn't be reading this book! Instead of giving the "right" answer, give the *real* answer – what is the worst thing you can imagine happening? People with gut problems often imagine all sorts of awful, and even catastrophic outcomes. For example, people foresee all kinds of negative social and work-related out-comes like: "My date will think I'm weird or disgusting"; "I'll have to leave the meeting and I'll be perceived as incompetent"; "I won't be able to get through the presentation"; "My friends will pity me and think I'm weak"; "I'll never be able to have a normal life." These are stressful thoughts! If they even cross your mind, your stress level will rise accordingly.

Now comes the challenging part! The next step is to identify some benign alternatives to the thoughts you have listed. Be careful not to simply contradict your negative predictions (e.g. by saying, "Maybe that won't happen.") The problem with such simple opposite statements is that they aren't very convincing. What you need to do is come up with an alternative scenario. For example, you might think to yourself, "If I disappear into the bathroom for a while, my date may wonder if I'm trying to ditch him. I could just tell him that there was a long line." In a work setting, you might consider the alternative that you could tolerate the gut distress for a period of time – it might calm down – and even if you do need to step out for a few minutes, no one will think that much of it as long as you present the information you were there to report.

The real key to giving these benign alternatives "teeth" – that is, making them more believable than your initial negative thoughts – is that you have to consider the *evidence* for and against each set of beliefs. For example, you might ask yourself what goes through your mind if you see someone else get up and leave a meeting for a few minutes. People often step out of meetings to go to the bathroom, refresh their coffee, answer a cell phone call or page, etc. Do you conclude that *they* are weird, pathetic, weak or incompetent? Probably not! Then what evidence do you have that other people are drawing those conclusions about you? Here's another example. If you found yourself thinking, "I can't stand this," a benign alternative might be that you have in fact tolerated GI symptoms in the past, even in situations where it was difficult. Or perhaps you can think of other types of discomfort that you have tolerated or survived. You may well be stronger and tougher than you think. While GI discomfort certainly isn't pleasant, it's not typically catastrophic either, especially if it's not the result of active disease. Of course you'd rather not experience those symptoms, but lots of people have to tolerate physical discomfort of all different kinds, like chronic back pain or arthritis. It's not fun. No one would choose it. But it's not the end of the world either. If you can manage to start thinking of GI symptoms as *uncomfortable and annoying* rather than as *painful and disabling* you might find them easier to tolerate. Is it fair that you have this problem? No. But it needn't be catastrophic either.

You may be wondering if this same advice applies during active flares. IBD flares almost always involve an increase in GI discomfort that can really only be described as painful. When I suggest downplaying that as "uncomfortable" you may feel invalidated and like I'm trivializing the very real pain you experience from time to time. Pain sucks. It's exhausting, distracting and very, very frustrating. But here's the thing. Losing days of your life, not getting to work, missing out on time with family and friends, sucks even more. I'm not asking you to be a superhero. There may be times when you simply need to stay home and take care of yourself. But remember, stress and distress amplify GI symptoms, especially abdominal pain, and ultimately, quality of life is more determined by the activities you engage in than by your level of physical discomfort. So there may well be times when you'll be tempted to opt out of life activities, but if you go ahead and do them anyway, you'll find you can enjoy yourself and might, actually, feel a little bit better. A benign alternative for you might be, "Well, sure, I'll be uncomfortable, but I'd rather be uncomfortable watching my daughter's concert than be uncomfortable and sad and angry that I missed it entirely. I won't be *more* uncomfortable if I go, and I will be unhappy if I don't go."

Here's a sample thought record that someone with an IBD might generate:

Situation	Thoughts	Feelings	Alternatives	Evidence
Went for a run for the first time in several months. Felt out of breath quickly and then felt very tired and sore for a few days afterwards	Oh no! What if this means my IBD is flaring again. Feeling so breathless and tired and sore probably means I'm anemic or malnourished or both. My gut must not be working right, not absorbing nutrients. This means I'm getting sick again. This is awful. My meds must not be working. I may have to try new meds that have more serious and scary side effects	Anxious Frustrated Upset Scared	Maybe I'm just out of shape Maybe I need to take it a little slower Maybe I felt tired and sore because I pushed it a little too hard the first time out	I haven't been running for several months. It makes sense that I would be out of shape. That explains feeling out of breath I did try to run three whole miles. Maybe that was unrealistic. If I think about what advice an athletic trainer would give to *anyone* who hadn't been exercising for a while, I realize I tried to do too much I remember being tired and sore after hard workouts in high school and college before this whole IBD thing even started If I'm just out of shape, it should get better every time I run If I'm really worried about the possibility of anemia or vitamin deficiencies, I can always get some blood work done to check

Here's another example.

Situation	Thoughts	Feelings	Alternatives	Evidence
I have to take part in a panel presentation at work next week. I'll be sitting up on stage with three other people in front of the whole audience	If my gut acts up it's going to be a *nightmare* Everyone's eyes will be on me I'll be *trapped* I won't be able to just get up and leave and go to the bathroom. It would be *bizarre* and incredibly *disruptive* Everyone will wonder what the heck is going on with me and the presentation will be a *disaster*	Anxious Panicky Frustrated Desperate	I won't be alone up there. If I need to step out my colleagues can take over for five to ten minutes If I tell my co-presenters that I may need to step out because I'm having GI issues, they will be understanding and they won't be surprised if it happens Most people in the audience may be curious for a few moments, but they'll be focused on the content, not on me personally I can pull out my cell phone as I get up to leave. People really do need to take emergency calls sometimes – no one in the audience needs to know it's a call of nature	I'm presenting with smart capable people. They can cover for me I don't think I've ever actually seen someone step away from a panel presentation – it will be odd and bit disruptive, but most people tend to just roll with stuff and won't be that curious or judgmental Even if it interrupts the flow of the presentation a little, having to excuse myself won't make it a *disaster* If my gut acts up, it wouldn't be ideal, but we can probably make it work

And another...

Situation	Thoughts	Feelings	Alternatives	Evidence
I'm dating this really nice person and I'd love to have them over to order dinner, watch a movie, and maybe even sleep over	What if my gut makes weird noises or I have diarrhea or I'm in so much pain I can't even enjoy the movie?	Anxious Panicky Frustrated Sad	If this person is really as kind and thoughtful as I think they are, I can just tell them I have some chronic GI issues and have to be careful what I eat. I could even tell them I have to use the rest room more often than most people	I've never actually been incontinent in bed. There's no reason to believe it will randomly happen tonight The kind of relationship I want is with someone who is generous and kind

Situation	Thoughts	Feelings	Alternatives	Evidence
	I'll have to keep interrupting the movie to go to the bathroom He/she will get really annoyed with me and it will be disruptive If he/she does spend the night, I'm terrified I will fart in bed, or worse, I might be incontinent I'm going to disgust them and humiliate myself It's probably better just to tell them I'll take a rain check and skip the whole thing		If he/she gets annoyed with me, it's a sign that they're not the right person for me. If they're understanding and sweet about it, that's a really good sign If I cancel the date I'll be sad and lonely and they'll think I don't like them, which is totally not the case, and would be worse than just being honest with them	I've cancelled things before and I always end up feeling sad and lonely and left out. The last person I was interested finally stopped calling because I flaked so often. I should try a different approach this time

Now you try. Refer back to the scenario you wrote about above in which you identified a situation, your thoughts and your feelings. Now enter some possible *benign alternatives* and the evidence for and against them.

Situation	Thoughts	Feelings	Alternatives	Evidence

Coming up with benign alternatives can be particularly difficult when the automatic thoughts are reflecting deeper, more core beliefs. For example, you might be having the automatic thought, "If I have GI symptoms, it is terrible and it will ruin my day." This might well be based on a deeper, core belief like, "If anything goes wrong, it ruins everything." In another example, you might think, "If I get flustered during the meeting because my gut is acting up, everyone will think I'm an idiot." This might be based on the core belief, "If I'm not perfect, then I'm a total failure." While these extreme, black and white thoughts may look silly in print, it's surprising how many folks believe them without even realizing they believe them!

Take a moment to ask yourself whether you hold any beliefs like this. Is it truly okay for you to make a mistake, or do you have trouble forgiving yourself? Does it matter if a few people don't like or respect you all that much? Is conflict intolerable to you, no matter what the situation? What if one person in a group *does* think you're incompetent, or gross, or weird? Is it impossible to take pleasure in an event or outing if things don't go perfectly? If you fail at one task or challenge, does that make *you* a failure? Is it unacceptable to fail?

As you learned in the last chapter, if your reactions to specific situations are driven by these kinds of core beliefs, then you have to address more than the negative automatic thoughts that are specific to the situation. You have to address the underlying core belief as well. One useful way to do this is to ask yourself what you would say to a close friend or loved one who expressed such a belief to you. Would you agree with them? Or would you argue with them? Most people hold themselves to much tougher (and more unrealistic!) standards than they hold other people. If your best friend or your child told you that they were a failure and that their life was ruined because they had screwed up one particular thing, what would you say? Now turn around and say the same thing to yourself! Why should different rules apply to you than to the rest of the people in your life? Only the gods are perfect. Real people make mistakes and have bad days. We're not liked and respected by everyone we know. A big part of this program is about learning to question extreme, unrealistic beliefs that set you up for stress and exacerbate your gut problems and make it harder to cope with life's challenges. If you can learn to do this, you are well on your way to reclaiming your life from your GI symptoms.

Suggested Activities

1   Continue to fill in thought records three to four times this week. Pay special attention to times when your gut was actually acting up or you were worried about IBD symptoms and the effect they might have on your social or work life.

2   Be sure to look for themes, watch out for core beliefs, and always to try to examine the evidence and consider things as objectively as possible.

Thought Record

Situation	Thoughts	Feelings	Alternatives	Evidence

Thought Record

Situation	Thoughts	Feelings	Alternatives	Evidence

Thought Record

Situation	Thoughts	Feelings	Alternatives	Evidence

6 Test It Out!

Behavioral Experiments

In the last chapter, I asked you to start applying the cognitive model directly to your thoughts about GI symptoms. For your homework, I asked you to complete another three to four thought records about situations in which your gut actually acted up. If you did the suggested activities, then you wrote about a few situations in which you were able to identify your thoughts and you discovered how your thoughts about the GI symptoms themselves may actually be contributing to further stress and distress and maybe even making the GI symptoms them-selves worse. Hopefully, you were able to come up with some *alternative* ways of thinking, and to examine the *evidence* for each set of thoughts to determine which was most likely to be true.

Sometimes, however, we simply don't have enough evidence to figure out the most accurate or objective way of looking at things. We may hold beliefs without having any evidence in one particular way or the other. For example, many people with gut problems believe that it is quite noticeable to other people when they have to excuse themselves to go to the bathroom. They don't really have any data or evidence to *support* this belief; they just assume it's true. On the other hand, when they think about it, they realize that they don't really have much data to contradict the belief either. In other words, they just don't have enough evidence in either direction to decide whether that belief is accurate or not.

If you find that you hold beliefs that you can't really support or contradict with evidence, then it's time to learn about *behavioral experiments*. Behavioral experiments are things you can do in the real world to gather *data* or *evidence* about beliefs. For example, suppose you are convinced that clambering over people in a row of chairs is just a terrible thing to do. It's impolite, disruptive, embarrassing and just generally not socially acceptable. Try to think of a way to gather data about this. For example, think of several different settings you could go spend time in, in which people are seated in rows – the movies, a place of worship, a PTA meeting, whatever. Now go to those settings, seat yourself where you can see most of the place (maybe even stand in back) and count how many people get up at some point and clamber over other people in their row. What would you predict? That no one does it? Or do a number of people do it at some point? Now, if possible, try to gauge the reactions of the people

DOI: 10.4324/9781003057635-7

being clambered over. Are they annoyed? Irritated? Put off? Or do people pretty much take this in stride and assume it's just a normal part of life? The results of such an experiment might surprise you.

Another approach to take would be to go to a movie theater, sit down, and then intentionally get up maybe half an hour into the movie and clamber over people. Go out of the theater, go back in, and sit in a different seat – climbing over people to get there. Do this again three or four times, slipping into different theaters so you're not climbing over the same people four or five times. Try to gauge the reactions of the people being climbed over. What would you predict? Would people huff and snort and roll their eyes? Or would they politely shift their legs and try to make room for you to get by? How do *you* feel if someone needs to slip past you in a row of seats? What do you conclude about them? If your beliefs about other people are basically benign, why do you think other people have negative beliefs about you?

Good behavioral experiments have several components, just like good scientific experiments. First, you have to have a hypothesis, or belief that you are putting to the test. Second, you need to set up a situation in which you can actually test the belief. Third, you have to have predictions about what will happen if the belief is true, versus what will happen if the belief is not true. Fourth, you have to actually go do the experiment and pay attention to what *actually* happens. Finally, you have to compare your prediction (what you thought would happen if your belief were true) to what actually happened (which may suggest that your original belief needs to be modified or changed).

For example, many people with gut problems believe that their friends would be grossed out, or would think they were weird or pathetic, if they knew about their "bathroom" issues. It's not hard to set up a situation in which you can test this belief – identify a close friend, someone you like and basically trust, who doesn't know about your gut problems, and explain to them a little bit about the difficulties you've been having. If your belief were true, you would *predict* that your friend would react in an awkward or unpleasant way. Perhaps at best they might change the subject very quickly without expressing much sympathy or concern or even curiosity. If your belief were *not* true, you would predict that your friend would react quite differently – expressing interest and concern and sympathy.

Now you have to go and tell your friend, and pay attention to how they *actually* react. This may feel very scary. You're taking a risk here. If your friend reacts well – that's great. You can start modifying your upsetting belief. But if your belief is true, and your friend reacts awkwardly or unpleasantly, you're stuck having told them. So ask yourself – what would be the worst thing about that? Maybe your friend reacted awkwardly because he or she just didn't know what to say. Maybe their opinion of you has actually changed – and for the worse. If that's the case, is this someone you *really* want to remain friends with? Good friends are understanding. Most people are sympathetic and flexible and just add new information to enrich their knowledge of someone. In the vast majority of cases, people actually feel *honored* to be taken into someone's confidence. It makes them feel closer to you because they know you trust them.

Many people will eventually return the honor by sharing more personal information with you. That's how friendships grow and deepen. So, while it's true that you might be taking a risk by carrying out this sort of behavioral experiment, you are also opening yourself up to the possibility of greater intimacy, trust and confidence in a friendship. If it doesn't work out – if the person you chose turns out to be unsympathetic, or laughs at you or is mean about it, you have a problem to solve – you need to find a better friend!

This exercise may be particularly anxiety provoking if you are someone who harbors a great deal of *shame* about your GI issues and has been working hard to keep your gut problems *secret*. Do you frequently make up "excuses" for having to skip social or work events involving food and drink? Do you worry a lot about what clients or co-workers or your boss or even friends and family will think about you using the bathroom frequently or having chronic diarrhea? Why? What are the underlying assumptions you're making here about how people would react if they knew "the truth?" Chances are, you're assuming that people would respond *much* more negatively than they actually would. If you present your condition in a straightforward, matter-of-fact way, people will generally take it in stride. Most people will be somewhat interested, genuinely concerned, and flattered that you told them. Many people will actually be *relieved* that there isn't something else going on. They may have thought that you didn't really like them all that much and that's why you wouldn't meet them for drinks or dinner – remember that other people catastrophize too!

I could share many examples from patients' lives about when they finally got up the courage to share the basics about their GI condition with someone and discovered, to their intense relief, that the person was pleased to know, thought better of them for having been straightforward, and worked with them to accommodate their need for more frequent bathroom visits, or different food or drink. Remember Mike, the businessman from the very beginning of the book, who had to travel frequently for work and came up with an endless variety of the "I must have had a bad burrito" stories to explain why he couldn't join his colleagues at restaurants or in the hotel bar after the day's work? He finally learned that telling people he had a "chronic GI condition" and so wouldn't be drinking, but would be happy to hang out for an hour after the meeting, was met with polite interest and occasional curiosity, and that most people simply said, "Glad you told me – see you at the bar!"

Another great example was from a woman with Crohn's who was actually working in a rehabilitation health care setting. She was very anxious about the possibility of having to walk out during a patient visit in order to use the bathroom. She ended up telling her supervisor, and they agreed to let patients know, very briefly and appropriately, that she might need to step out on occasion because of a GI related medical issue of her own. To her delight and surprise, not only were her co-workers supportive, but many of her patients told her how *inspired* they were by her – they saw her as professional and caring and effective and it gave them hope that they could overcome their own medical issues and live an equally satisfying and productive life.

Finally, a young woman with a history of UC, who had undergone a resection operation (but not a full J pouch procedure), was terribly embarrassed by her frequent need to fart, and terrified that she would pass stool without realizing it. She was very reluctant to have her boyfriend spend the evening with her watching a movie because every time she felt the need to pass gas, she would excuse herself to go to the bathroom. She was also terrified of letting him sleep over, afraid she would fart in her sleep, or worse experience incontinence in bed during sex or even while she was asleep. Ironically, the stress about all this just made her feel even gassier when he was around. She finally found the courage to tell him about the problem, and they agreed to just fart around each other. He told her it had improved *his* life a thousand percent, and it was fabulous to be able to feel so comfortable and easy in each other's company. She in turn said that this one change – feeling free to fart around him – had changed her life. She was thrilled the first time he slept over and she was able to relax enough to actually sleep through the night in the same bed.

So if you are one of those people who has been keeping your GI issues secret from people around you, now is the time to try a behavioral experiment to see what would really happen if you just told people. Don't make a big deal of it. It doesn't have to be a dramatic revelation. Just pick someone you feel reasonably comfortable with and, when you have an opportunity, let them know that you have a chronic GI condition that sometimes causes gut upset, and that you have to watch what you eat and/or make more frequent bathroom trips. Some people won't want to know any more. Many people may be curious and they may want to know more. Tell them as much as you feel comfortable revealing. Keep it light, factual and straightforward. If it feels right, use humor. Acknowledge that sometimes it's frustrating or limiting, but you make the best of it and try not to let it interfere with life. Then pay attention to how they react. Do any of your dire predictions come true? Or does the person react kindly and genuinely? You might very well be pleasantly surprised!

To summarize, in a behavioral experiment you want to:

1 *Identify* the negative belief you want to test and think of relevant situations you could set up that would let you test the belief.
2 *Predict* what will happen if the belief is true and consider what might happen if the belief is not true.
3 *Gather data* by carrying out the experiment and pay attention to what *actually* happens, even if this feels scary or seems to entail some "risk."
4 *Compare* what actually happened with what you predicted. What does the evidence suggest about your original belief?

Another example of a behavioral experiment is to test the belief that if you're having an active flare, you simply can't risk going out and about – to the mall or the movies or even to run errands. You may truly need frequent and urgent access to rest rooms, and you may believe that it is simply too "risky" or embarrassing to be out and about and need quick access to a bathroom. Recall that many states in the US actually have Restroom Access Acts (Ally's Laws) in place to ensure that people with medical conditions like IBDs can have access to rest room facilities in public places and retail establishments. Moreover, the CCF and many doctors' offices provide wallet-sized cards that are sufficient medical documentation of your medical need. Crohn's and Colitis UK will also issue "Can't Wait" cards in English and many other languages so that you can travel with them. If you have trouble believing you could ask to use a restroom in an emergency, this is a *great* behavioral experiment to try. Go out intentionally to a place where a public restroom is not typically available (the bank, a pharmacy chain store, a dry cleaner) and (at a time when you *don't* actually urgently need to use the restroom) ask to use the restroom as a matter of a medical emergency and *see what happens*. I suggested in Chapter 2 that the vast majority of people are truly kind, sympathetic and helpful. If you simply say, "I'm so sorry, but I need to use your restroom – it's a medical emergency," almost everyone will smile and show you the way. If you run into someone who is hesitant or skeptical, you can produce the card to back up your request. It's a good idea to try this experiment at a time when you don't actually need to go so that you can focus on the person's actual response. Try it at a few different establishments and see what happens.

You may run into a few people who give you a hard time. It may feel embarrassing to push the point. But part of this exercise is learning how to advocate for yourself in a straightforward and appropriately assertive way. If you try this, you'll find that *almost* everyone is quick to help and is understanding and accommodating without being overly curious or intrusive. You may get a hard "no" at some places. It's important to interpret it correctly. Don't assume they think you're inappropriate, and don't be embarrassed for having asked. Maybe the bank is set up in such a way that allowing the public access to their staff rest room would actually compromise security in some way. Maybe the supermarket staff bathroom is in the basement behind the industrial box baling machine and it truly wouldn't be safe to allow the public down there. (Most Restroom Access Acts do include exclusions for situations in which it would be an obvious health or safety risk to the customer or an obvious security risk to the retail establishment.) Hopefully they will be appropriately apologetic and will help you problem solve about where else you might go. Also be careful not to make negative assumptions about the people who say no. Many lower-level employees in customer service won't feel empowered to make decisions that run counter to general store policies.

On the other hand, if you run into someone who is truly nasty about it – unsympathetic, dismissive, rude and unhelpful – then you've learned never to visit that particular business again! In the US you can easily write a negative Yelp or Google review (with or without specifics) about the poor customer service and mistreatment of someone with a medical emergency. Businesses *hate* getting reviews like that, and might well reach out to you, especially if it's a smaller business, not a large national chain. It could be a real teachable moment for the employee in question, and you will have done the world a favor. This kind of self-advocacy can feel very empowering, even if it does take some energy and some courage to do it. Of course, you don't *have* to do this kind of advocacy if you don't have time or energy for it. You could just cross that business off your list of places to patronize. But don't let an experience like this defeat you. Think firmly that this was poor behavior on the part of the business's employee and remind yourself that they *should* have responded more positively. Then go to a competitor's business and see how they respond to the same sort of request. There is no need to feel embarrassed or defeated. Just annoyed and justified.

Another option to consider is keeping an "emergency" package in your car or backpack or tote bag. Such a package might include a travel pack of flushable wet wipes, a change of underwear, or even a spare pair of pants. Chances are good that you won't need it, even if you are having a mild to moderate flare, but taking it along might allow you to take "risks" and go places and do things you wouldn't do otherwise.

Behavioral medicine experts have known for years that some people with chronic diseases are quite disabled by them, while other people *with equal disease severity* seem to live fuller, happier lives. What's the difference? It isn't that the people in that second group are somehow "tougher" or "stronger" or have higher pain tolerance. It's that they choose to live fully despite having some limitations. So, if you would normally avoid going shopping or to a theater or your child's sporting event or recital during a flare, *go anyway*, even if you do end up sitting in the back, by the aisle and scoping out bathrooms first. If that's what it takes to get you out the door, then do it and *go*! Bring a change of underwear if you must, but don't miss out on life.

Remember that the purpose of all the cognitive work I introduced you to in Chapters 4 and 5 was *not* to put rose-colored glasses on. I don't want you to trade in a depressing or anxiety-provoking world view for a falsely optimistic world view. What I want is for you to be able to evaluate your beliefs *objectively* in light of the evidence, even if the evidence ends up convincing you of something that might be frustrating.

For example, imagine that you, like many people with an IBD, get up extra early in the morning to ensure that you have enough time for multiple trips to the bathroom (or one long session). You resent it every time your alarm clock goes off and you wonder if you're just being foolish getting up that early. Maybe you really don't need all that extra time. Wouldn't it be nice to feel *normal* and not have such a complicated morning ritual? You decide to try an experiment and see if you can sleep in later (getting another precious hour of shut-eye) without it affecting your gut. You try it the next day, and it *doesn't* go well. Because you feel rushed and stressed in the morning, you don't really have enough time to finish defecating in a peaceful, patient way. As a result, your gut is uncomfortable and crampy all morning. You end up having a few bloody, loose, urgent bowel movements later in the day.

What have you learned? Well, obviously the experiment did not allow you to conclude that you can sleep in later and have a "normal" morning. That would have been nice, but it isn't reality. At least not when your disease is active. You really need that extra hour of time at home to make multiple bathroom trips and finish defecating before you start your day. Ideally, what you *have* learned is that you have actually developed a routine that works pretty well for you and allows you to maximize your GI health and comfort. You might still resent having to get up early, but you can do so moving forward knowing that you are doing what is necessary to take care of yourself.

A terrific next step would be to find ways to make that necessary bathroom time feel self-nurturing. Lots of busy people get up earlier than "necessary" to nurse their coffee, read the paper, watch the sun come up, or just have some quiet moments to themselves to ease into the day before the rush of obligations starts. What if you used that necessary bathroom time to do a crossword or sudoku puzzle? You could use it to spend guilt-free time on Facebook or reading the news or playing a game on your phone. What if you had a great novel that you only got to read during that time? Is there a way to make that time feel like self-care, rather than a frustrating waste of time imposed on you by your disease? If so, then I would declare it a very successful behavioral experiment, even though it didn't ultimately provide the evidence that you were hoping for.

The problem with straight cognitive interventions is that lots of times we just don't have the evidence we need to know whether our initial negative beliefs are right or not. We may be able to come up with benign alternatives, but without the evidence to convince us, it may not help much. That's where behavioral experiments come in. They are clever ways of gathering data to help us decide which beliefs are valid and which ones aren't. Sometimes a behavioral experiment can be as simple as asking someone what they think. Of course, you have to trust that they will tell you the truth, and you have to be a little cautious about asking some people certain things. For example, I wouldn't necessarily ask my CEO if farting at meetings is problematic. But I might ask a trusted family member or very close friend how much they actually notice my farting and how much they care. If they know you want to hear the truth, they'll probably tell you. And honestly, our own body noises and emanations are much more obvious to us than to other people. So if your friend tells you that they have no idea what you're talking about and have never noticed you farting more than anyone else, believe them!

Other times behavioral experiments have to be more subtle or more clever, or you may have to set up situations that will allow you to test certain beliefs. Sometimes you can gather data about other people just by watching them, like the movie theater example in which you simply count the number of times other people get up and climb over others during a movie.

Sometimes behavioral experiments can feel very scary. It's always a good idea to pick something to do initially that feels "do-able" so that even if the outcome isn't what you hoped for (maybe your girlfriend tells you that she does notice your farts and gut rumblings and doesn't exactly think they're attractive) you still have someplace positive to go with it (after all, she loves you anyway, and isn't going anywhere, so maybe it doesn't matter all that much). The more you can incorporate behavioral experiments into your life, the less likely it is that unfounded negative thoughts will continue to control your emotional life and the better off you will be.

Suggested Activities

1   Try to think of one behavioral experiment you could do this week that would provide some real data about a negative belief you hold.

Belief I am testing:

Behavioral experiment I can do to test it:

What would happen if my belief were *true*?

What would happen if my belief were *not true*?

What *actually* happened?

How should I modify my belief to take this new evidence into account?

---

1   Continue to do thought records two to three times a week. The situations don't have to be "big" – anything that caused you the least twinge of stress or anxiety will work. The point is to keep practicing these skills until they become second nature.

Thought Record

Situation	Thoughts	Feelings	Alternatives	Evidence

Thought Record

Situation	Thoughts	Feelings	Alternatives	Evidence

Thought Record

Situation	Thoughts	Feelings	Alternatives	Evidence

7 Eliminating Avoidance

In this chapter, I'm going to switch gears a little bit, and start talking about avoidance – something *lots* of people with gut problems are very good at!

Avoidance is a perfectly natural and often adaptive coping strategy. In fact, if we didn't learn to avoid things that were bad for us, we wouldn't live very long! The first time you get a burn, you learn to *avoid* touching hot things. If you know something is dangerous, you *should* avoid it! Unfortunately, humans often avoid things for the wrong reasons, and avoiding things you don't really need to avoid is usually a pretty bad idea.

Here are some examples of common, but maladaptive, avoidance behaviors.

1 *Procrastination.* People often avoid doing things because they are anxious about them. They think things like "I hate this. It's overwhelming. It will be too hard or too unpleasant. I won't be able to do it. It'll feel awful. I'll be bad at it. Even if I do it, it'll turn out badly." Sound familiar? Everyone procrastinates sometimes. The problem with procrastination, of course, is that it ultimately makes you feel worse. Now you still have the task to do, and you feel guilty and even more anxious on top of it because you let it go too long! Most of the time, once we actually sit ourselves down to do the task, it turns out to be much easier and less painful than we were anticipating. One useful trick is to make a deal with yourself – sit down and work on it for five to ten minutes. If it really feels awful, you can stop. In the vast majority of cases, you find it's really not that bad, and you just keep working!
2 *Phobic avoidance.* People with phobias of specific things (like elevators or dogs or spiders) often go to great lengths to avoid coming into contact with the thing they're scared of. It can get to the point where it really interferes with life. The problem with avoidance is that people never have the chance to learn that the thing they're so scared of really isn't that dangerous.
3 *Social avoidance.* This is a big one for a lot of people. In some people, this is severe enough to be diagnosed as social anxiety disorder. But *lots* of people have mild social avoidance. Maybe they hate speaking up in class or in meetings. Maybe they have to have a drink or two every time they go to a party to take the edge off their anxiety so they can relax enough to have a

DOI: 10.4324/9781003057635-8

decent time. Even though the person went to the party, drinking to numb the anxiety is still avoidance. It's obvious how this could get in your way professionally or socially. What's less obvious is that avoidance actually makes anxiety *worse*. You become more and more convinced that you *can't* do the things you avoid doing. As a result, they get scarier and scarier, and you never have the chance to learn new skills or to realize that you actually can do these things.

People with gut problems typically avoid a number of things for reasons that *look* perfectly sensible on the face of them. The problem with this is that it can really limit your life and make things less fun and less productive. Once you start avoiding a few things, it gets more and more tempting to avoid lots of things. If you have started to avoid things because of your GI symptoms, you probably already know that this isn't working out that well for you. You may have escaped or avoided a few stressful things in the short run, but in the long run, your life isn't better because you're avoiding things, it's worse. The bottom line is that

AVOIDANCE DOESN'T WORK.

Here's a list of the sorts of things people with gut problems often avoid.

Visceral Sensations

Most people with gut problems are both hypersensitive to visceral (or gut) sensations and hypervigilant about them. Because you may fear the onset of GI symptoms, you may monitor your body for signs of an impending flare. People with secondary IBS in particular will often go to great lengths to avoid experiencing those sensations if at all possible. They view *any* abdominal discomfort as intolerable – painful, debilitating, incapacitating – and to be avoided whenever possible by whatever means necessary. This leads to avoidance of lots of other things (tight clothing that presses on the abdomen, possible "trigger" foods and stressful situations) and to reactive use of medications (like anti-diarrheal drugs) in a futile attempt to fend off any and all abdominal discomfort. It also leads to retreating from life experiences, opportunities and challenges (say to curl up in bed with a heating pad pressed to the tummy). One of the most important things you can do to help yourself overcome the disabling aspects of gut problems is to stop thinking of *all* GI sensations as heralding painful attacks that make you sick and must be avoided at all costs. Some GI sensations are just uncomfortable, annoying and occasionally inconvenient. *Everyone* experiences uncomfortable visceral sensations from time to time. Yours are undoubtedly worse and more frequent, which isn't fair or fun, but it's not necessarily catastrophic either. It's quite unrealistic to avoid all visceral sensations. Assuming that your IBD is being well managed medically, if you can learn that not all twinges, cramps or gurgles are dangerous, and many visceral sensations can be acknowledged and then safely ignored (like the smoke detector that goes off every time you boil water), you'll be well on your way to taking back control of your life.

Of course, if you are in the middle of an active flare, then you may *need* to track your symptoms and be in touch with your doctor. Sometimes burning pain signals a true recurrence of inflammation that needs to be managed more aggressively. Sometimes acute abdominal pain can signal a condition (like a small bowel obstruction or a fistula) that really *does* need medical attention. In severe cases, such things could even require emergency intervention. The key for people with an IBD is to learn to tell the difference between sensations that signal a real problem and sensations that can safely be ignored. If you've required surgery in the past, or experienced medical complications or emergencies with your IBD, you are especially likely to be hypervigilant about abdominal discomfort. The more objective you can be about understanding different sensations and levels of discomfort, and learning which ones are important and which ones probably aren't, the better off you'll be. Talk to your physician about when it is important to seek medical attention, and when you can safely delay or ignore attending to visceral sensations.

Food

People with gut problems develop all kinds of beliefs about which foods do or do not upset them. Some of the most commonly cited "no-no" foods include coffee, dairy, meat, wheat, fruit, fried, greasy or spicy foods, carbonated beverages, chocolate, alcohol, salad greens and raw veggies and beans. People with IBDs often try various restrictive diets, eliminating gluten, or dairy. Some even commit to the low FODMAP diet, one of the most restrictive diets of all. People with IBDs may indeed have to make specific dietary changes *during acute flares* (especially avoiding high residue foods like nuts, popcorn, celery and whole tomatoes), but there is very little data suggesting that those changes need to be maintained when not having an active flare. There's no question that different foods affect digestive processes differently and you should, of course, follow your doctor's advice for managing your diet safely. (See Chapter 8 for a detailed discussion of diet and nutrition in inflammatory bowel diseases.)

But people with IBDs, and especially people with secondary IBS, sometimes develop significant *fear of food*. Food starts to feel dangerous and eating starts to feel like a gamble that may well result in pain and urgency. Take a moment to complete the Fear of Food Questionnaire in Appendix C to see if this applies to you.

If you are afraid of food you may have developed all kinds of strategies for managing your diet to the point where it becomes difficult to keep track of it all, and some or most of it may not be necessary or even helpful. I worked with one woman with Crohn's who was so anxious about food that she would *only* eat pureed baby food – even when she wasn't in flare. (She particularly liked Beechnut chicken and rice and Gerber's pureed sweet potato and banana.) Needless to say, this highly restrictive and fairly unappealing diet really wasn't appropriate for an adult, and it was quite expensive! Sometimes people get so anxious about whether a food might cause pain or diarrhea that they develop *superstitious* avoidance. Say you once ate a small apple or a few table-spoons of hummus and later that night or even the next day your gut acted up. You might conclude that you should never eat apple or hummus again. But what if your gut acted up for totally different reasons – say because you had a stressful meeting coming up? Then you're denying yourself a perfectly nutritious, benign and delicious food for no good reason! If you have been avoiding or severely limiting a number of foods – *even when you're not in flare* – you need to read Chapter 8, which covers the scientific evidence about diet. But before you read Chapter 8, take a moment to reflect on what you currently believe about food and your GI symptoms, and list foods you typically avoid or restrict.

Beliefs about food:

Foods I avoid or restrict:

The most extreme form of avoidance of food is *fasting*. Lots of people with IBDs avoid *eating* during the day all together. They skip breakfast and lunch and then only eat dinner (and maybe a snack) when they're back in the safety of their own home at the end of the day. After all, if you don't eat, there won't be anything in your gut and you won't have to deal with pain or urgency or having to go to the bathroom. This is a problematic strategy for any number of reasons.

First of all, not eating on any particular day is going to make you *hungry*. This sounds obvious and trivial, but sometimes people don't truly think through all the implications of this. Being hungry means lots of things are going on physiologi-cally. Perhaps most importantly, you are going to end up hypoglycemic – that is with low blood sugar. Glucose (blood sugar) is the essential fuel that powers all the cells in the human body, including muscle and brain cells. Hunger leads to:

- Weakness
- Fatigue
- Dizziness
- Tremor

- Impaired coordination
- Slowed reaction time
- Irritability
- Anxiety
- Poor problem solving
- Low frustration tolerance
- Impaired attention
- Impaired concentration
- Impaired memory

If that were the list of side effects a medication was almost guaranteed to cause, would you take it? Probably not! Unless it was actually a life-saving and necessary treatment, you'd probably tell your doctor, "No way!" But that's what you're subjecting yourself to when you skip breakfast and lunch in order to avoid the possibility of GI distress later in the day.

The second problem with not eating is that in the long term you are compromising the nutrition and calories your body needs to function, keep itself healthy, and repair itself from damage. Different countries, ethnic regions and cultures emphasize different meals and load calories at different times, but *all* human cuisines include multiple meals during the day. This makes sense, because humans are omnivores who evolved from foragers, and foragers typically need to eat quite frequently. (Large carnivorous hunters like lions and wolves typically eat much less frequently. They can gorge on large amounts of meat when they kill something and then go for several days just digesting and gnawing on bones.) Unlike lions and wolves, however, humans can't fill all their nutritional needs in a single meal. We just can't eat enough. Getting adequate nutrition (and maintaining a healthy body weight) is often challenging for people with IBDs. Your ability to *absorb* nutrients and calories from food may already be compromised. Your gut will have a much easier time extracting what it needs if the food comes in smaller quantities more regularly. So for all of these reasons, avoiding eating is probably not a great idea.

Food Situations

Another category of things people with gut problems often prefer to avoid are various *situations* that are likely to involve food and eating. This obviously includes restaurants, but also includes parties, being invited out to people's homes for meals, social events at bars or clubs, any place where there is likely to be social eating and/or drinking, and where it might be awkward or embarrassing to refuse certain foods, ask for special foods, or have gut problems related to particular foods.

In the box below, go ahead and list any food situations that you might avoid. Note if you always avoid them, sometimes avoid them, occasionally avoid them, or wish you could avoid them, even though you don't.

Food situations I prefer to avoid

Situations Where Bathrooms are Hard to Find

The final category of things people with gut problems often prefer to avoid are situations in which you might get stuck in some way, especially places where it might be hard to get to a bathroom, or where people would notice if you got up and left. Common situations that people with GI symptoms tend to avoid include:

Various things related to transportation:

- Long car trip
- Subway
- Train
- Bus
- Airplane
- Elevator
- Bridge/tunnel

Situations in which many people sit in rows:

- Places of worship
- Movie theaters
- Concerts or shows
- Sports stadiums
- Classes

Crowded public places or places where you might get stuck in line:

- Supermarkets
- Zoos
- Amusement parks
- Airport security

Places or situations where bathrooms are hard to find or hard to get to:

- Playground
- Beach
- Camping
- Skiing
- Outdoor vacations
- Outdoor concerts or events
- Shopping malls

Work situations in which leaving might be difficult or awkward:

- Meetings
- Conferences
- Presentations
- Conference calls
- Front desk/reception

In the box below, please list the places or situations you generally prefer to avoid. Of course, this may vary depending on whether you're in flare or not, or even depending on how your gut has been acting over the last few days or even that morning. If you had a "good" morning it might not worry you to go out to a movie, but if it's been a bad few days, you might be very reluctant to go. You can note that too. If you really don't avoid anything, good for you! Just note that you don't avoid things. If you *do* avoid things, do your best to list the situations *in order of difficulty*. That is, list the places you would always avoid, if possible, or tolerate only with extreme difficulty first, then go down in difficulty until you get to places you'd sometimes prefer to avoid, but can tolerate okay even on a bad day. Next to each place or situation, I'd also like you to rate how much distress you think it would cause you if you had to do it. Use a scale from 0–100, where: 100 is horrendous, intolerable anxiety, stress and upset – the worst you've ever experienced; 60 or 70 is really awful – really hard to tolerate, although you could suck it up for a very short period of time; 40 or 50 is pretty bad; 20 or 30 isn't much fun, but you could definitely tolerate it if you had to; 10 is just a bit of discomfort, "normal" anxiety or a tiny bit of gut distress. This is called a *subjective unit of distress* (or SUD) score. There's nothing magical about it. You could rate things from 1–10, or 0–7, or whatever you wanted. We usually use 0–100 because it provides lots of ratings in the middle of the scale. Do your best to order the things on your list so that the distress rating starts really high and goes down pretty low, with a few things in the middle of the rating scale as well. Also be sure you have some items that are really low on the list, things you could do with only minimal discomfort.

Situations you prefer to avoid	SUD score
Things it would be *extremely* difficult or even impossible to do:	80–100
Things it would be *quite* difficult to tolerate:	60–79
Things it would be *moderately* difficult to do:	40–59
Things you could do that would be *uncomfortable* but feel manageable:	20–39
Things you could do with only *minimal* discomfort or anxiety	0–19

Subtle Avoidance

The last category of things people with gut problems often avoid may not sound like avoidance to you at all. I call it *subtle* avoidance because although it looks like you're engaging in activities and going places, you're really still doing things to avoid the *possibility* of embarrassment, discomfort or distress related to GI symptoms.

One particularly pernicious type of subtle avoidance that a few IBD patients get caught in is using anti-anxiety medications from the benzodiazepine group. These include Valium (diazepam), Klonopin (clonazepam), Ativan (lorazepam), Librium (chlordiazepoxide) and Xanax (alprazolam). This class of drugs is particularly seductive because they provide very fast relief from feelings of anxiety and stress, and may actually make secondary GI distress calm down as well. Unfortunately, they come with a host of problems. First of all, they have cognitive side effects. They can make you feel a little out of it or sleepy, and they affect reaction time and memory. They are also not meant to be used long term because our brains develop *tolerance* to them. This means either that the usual dose stops working or that you have to take more over time to get the same effect. (Benzos mimic a naturally occurring brain chemical or neurotransmitter called GABA. GABA is an inhibitory chemical that stops a lot of the processes involved in sympathetic activation. When you take a benzo long term, the brain stops making as much naturally occurring GABA because it senses all this "fake" GABA floating around. As your own production of GABA goes down, you'll need more fake GABA – that is a higher dose of the benzo – to get the same effect.) This biological process also leads to *withdrawal* and rebound anxiety if you try to stop the medication. Take away the daily dose of fake GABA, and your brain is now a quart low on real GABA – you'll end up *more* anxious than you would have been if you had never taken the medication to begin with.

Even if you use a benzo only once in while, just when you're feeling particularly anxious, they can still get in the way of true recovery. Sometimes people carry around a few doses of a benzo just "in case" they need it. They may never even use any of it, but just carrying it around with them makes them feel more secure. It's not at all obvious to many people why this is problematic. The reason is that you are still thinking about things in a catastrophic way. If the only thing standing between you and perceived potential disaster is the pill in your pocket, you're still dependent on it, even if you hardly ever use it. It keeps you from learning how resilient and competent you are and how you can get through discomfort and anxiety. The more you practice that, the less discomfort and anxiety you will experience.

Another thing people with IBDs do is use anti-diarrheal medications *reactively*. There are a number of medications that can be used to treat the most disruptive symptoms of IBDs. These include Questran (cholestyramine) and Colestid (colestipol). Both of these medications lower cholesterol and reduce bile acid. Both of them have *constipation* as a "side effect" and they are pretty effective anti-diarrheals that are often prescribed to people with IBDs. Additionally, some people with Crohn's have bile acid malabsorption/excess bile acid, resulting in bile acid diarrhea, particularly after surgery to remove the lower part of the small intestine. These medications are also effective treatments for that. Other anti-diarrheal drugs that your doctor may approve of using include the over-the-counter drug Imodium (loperamide) and the prescription drug Lomotil (diphenoxylate and atropine). It is absolutely appropriate to use these medications to manage urgency and watery diarrhea *if* your doctor has given you the green light. One problem arises when people start "chasing" their symptoms and end up over correcting. This can lead to unfortunate cycles of diarrhea and constipation.

For example, your doctor may suggest taking a single dose of colestipol daily, or up to as many as four. If you have diarrhea and urgency one day, you may be tempted to take three or four colestipol the next day to try to prevent further diarrhea. You may then end up slightly constipated, and need to skip the colestipol all together the following day and take extra fiber supplements (like Metamucil or Citrucel) to get things moving. Indeed, especially for individuals with strictures or a post-surgical anastomosis, constipation can be risky. Rather than swinging from one extreme to another in a desperate effort to avoid or prevent GI symptoms, a much better strategy is to make *small* changes day to day and experiment with consistent dosing strategies. For example, it might make sense to try taking a single colestipol and a teaspoon of Citrucel every morning. If your gut is acting up, try taking *two* colestipol the next day. In other words, don't over-react. The gut is a dynamic system that responds to changes both acutely and over time. If you make dramatic, slightly panicky adjustments to your medication in response to acute symptoms, you may actually exacerbate your difficulties chronically.

Another problem that can arise is when people try to micromanage their stools and GI sensations. One patient with Crohn's I worked with used to keep a daily diary of her GI symptoms and bowel movements. She kept this diary for *years*. Very occasionally it was helpful in establishing her response to a new IBD medication regimen. But she continued to keep the diary even when she was medically stable. She would then make all kinds of small adjustments to various medications (often against her doctor's advice) in an attempt to control exactly what was going on in her gut and coming out of it. She actually made so many changes, she could never tell which change caused what. She spent huge amounts of time and energy tracking her stools and what she ate and adjusting various meds differently every day. I strongly suggested that she *stop* keeping the diary (this made her very anxious at first) and that she stop making so many adjustments to her medications. Her attempts to control her gut functioning (and thus *avoid* any sensations or stool issues that concerned her) were back-firing and keeping her anxious and overly focused on her IBD. She finally settled into a regimen that was consistent, but had some flexibility. She took her neuromodulator every day at the dose recommended by her doctor, she took two colestipol every evening with dinner, and if she had diarrhea in the morning, she would take a single Imodium before breakfast. If she didn't have a bowel movement at all one day, she would take a single colestipol at dinner that night. This strategy was very effective, and she stopped spending so much time and energy tracking every symptom, second guessing her doctors and trying to micromanage both her medications and her GI functioning.

Obviously if a medication has been prescribed by your doctor and you are supposed to be using it in a particular way as part of your medical management strategy, then follow your doctor's advice. But if you're uncertain about the value, safety or appropriate use of a particular medication, be sure to check with your doctor so you understand what it's for and why and when and how you're supposed to use it.

If you do engage in these or any other "subtle" avoidance behaviors, please list them below. As you did above, try to list them in order, so that the things it would be most anxiety provoking to give up are listed at the top, and things that are the least important to you, or would be the least difficult to give up, are listed at the bottom. Be sure to give each one a SUD score that represents the degree of distress you think you'd experience if you tried to give up that behavior.

Subtle avoidance strategies	SUD score
Things it would be *extremely* difficult or even impossible to give up:	80–100
Things it would be *quite* difficult to give up:	60–79
Things it would be *moderately* difficult to give up:	40–59
Things you could give up that would feel *uncomfortable* but bearable:	20–39
Things you could give up with only *minimal* discomfort or anxiety:	0–19

Now, let's acknowledge that when you've been avoiding things, it's no good at all telling you to "just do it." Your friends and family may have tried this, in which case you know it isn't helpful. In fact, it can actually make things worse. Here's how it often unfolds. Imagine that you force yourself to "suck it up" and try going somewhere or doing something that makes you really anxious. Maybe you can endure it for a short time, but it gets overwhelming and you leave. Or you endure it for a while and your gut acts up so much that you have an awful experience. Either way, you have probably *sensitized* yourself to the situation. That is, you've basically confirmed that it was awful, and that you probably *should* have avoided it in the first place. You may even be *more* anxious about it from now on. Not good! And definitely not what we're going for here. You need some other strategy to help you overcome avoidance.

If you are avoiding situations or places, it's time to introduce you to the concept of *exposure therapy*. Exposure therapy is based on some very straightforward principles of learning, and there is *tons* of evidence that it works. The basic logic behind exposure therapy is that you have to expose yourself *slowly*. When you carve things up into little, manageable chunks, it's much easier to do them. Approaching the problem of avoidance this way is much gentler and it's much more likely to be successful. Eventually, exposure therapy lets you handle things that would be awful if you tried them right away with only minimal discomfort and anxiety. Let's look at a fairly straightforward example of exposure therapy in action with a very specific problem – fear of snakes.

Imagine for a moment that you were really creeped out by snakes. (This probably won't be hard. Most people in the world really don't like snakes much. In fact, most *primates* really don't like snakes much!) But now imagine that it's so bad that it interferes with your life. You won't go for a walk in the woods or even do any gardening because you might encounter a snake. You freak out if a television show or movie shows a snake, or if you come across a picture of a snake in a magazine. What would you normally do? Avoid them! Even to the point of quickly changing the channel or closing the magazine. What does that avoidance do? Sensitizes you! You see the picture or image, your heart thuds, you feel a little squirt of adrenaline, you quickly get rid of the image, and then you start to feel less scared. You've just told your brain, "Wow! That was scary and dangerous! Good thing I got away from it!" This just seems to confirm that snakes are really threatening and should be avoided at all costs.

In exposure therapy, the first thing we do is have someone construct an *anxiety hierarchy*. This is just a fancy term for a list of things that scare them from most scary to least scary. The scariest thing for a snake phobic person would probably be trying to wrap a live snake around their neck. The least scary thing might be looking at a small picture of a very young, harmless snake. There would probably be lots of things in the middle, including looking at a caged snake in a zoo, putting their hand up to the glass of the cage, taking the lid off the cage of a harmless pet snake, touching the snake with one finger while the snake was being held by someone else, and so on. Each of these things could be rated on a scale from 0 (none at all) to 100 (the worst, most intense feeling possible) in terms of how scary or anxiety provoking it would be.

The next step would be for the person to *expose* themselves to the lowest ranked thing on the hierarchy. This might be a benign picture of a little baby garden snake. It might cause about 20 SUD units of anxiety. The trick is – and this is important – that the person would need to *keep looking* at the picture until their discomfort began to go away. This is technically called *habituation*. It basically means that your brain gets bored of the stimulus. You can only stare at a picture for so long without realizing that nothing bad is actually happening. It might take five minutes, or 20 minutes, but eventually the picture just stops being scary, and the person's SUD rating drops to between 0 and 5.

Now here's the beautiful part. The *next* thing on the hierarchy, say walking into a room with a caged snake 15 feet away, might originally have been about a 30 or 35 on the anxiety hierarchy. But once the picture no longer feels scary, walking into the room only feels like about a 20 on the SUD scale. Sure, the person's anxiety goes back up, but not as high as it would have if walking into the room was the first thing they had done. Again, you just have the person sit by the door until their discomfort begins to subside. Snakes are actually pretty boring. They just lie under a log almost all the time. Watching a snake in a cage is a lot like watching paint drying. Booorrring! So eventually, your brain stops sending "DANGER!" messages and encodes that nothing much is really going on here. You've learned that this isn't so terrible, you can handle the distress, and you don't really need to avoid this level of contact with snakes after all.

And like magic, the next thing on the list drops down in terms of how anxiety provoking it will feel. It's as if you had a stack of wooden blocks, and every time you pull one out from the bottom, the higher ones all drop down a level too. This goes on, step by step, until eventually you find that you have worked your way all the way up to the top of the hierarchy! But the amazing thing is that by the time you actually pick up the snake yourself, it only causes about 25–30 SUD units of anxiety. If you had just tried it off the bat, it would have been up at 100, and you wouldn't have been able to tolerate it. People sometimes mistakenly think that the goal of exposure therapy is to get them to tolerate extreme distress. Nothing could be further from the truth. When done well, exposure therapy *never* results in discomfort much higher than about a 30 (somewhere in the moderate but definitely tolerable range) on the person's SUD scale. Not much fun, perhaps, but not difficult to endure, especially since it tends to come down pretty quickly.

Now the good news is that you've already done the first step – you created your anxiety hierarchies earlier on in this chapter! Hopefully this was useful in and of itself. Just creating the anxiety hierarchy often helps people realize that not all situations are equally horrible or difficult to tolerate. Sometimes when we're anxious, we tend to lump all related situations into one big scary, undoable blob. Teasing that blob apart into more and less anxiety provoking steps helps you realize that you really can do more than you might think.

Your homework this week is to focus on two situations that you avoid or prefer to avoid, or two examples of subtle avoidance. Pick two of the easiest things, the ones lowest on your SUD scale, preferably not more than about 25 "units" of distress, and *go do them*. Depending on how avoidant you tend to be, it might be something as small as "drive around the block a bunch of times" or as big as "take the train into the city." The key is to make sure you do it long enough for your anxiety to come down from a high of about 25 to at most a 10, or better yet 5 or even 0. As long as your anxiety is on the way *down* you can stop doing it. If the thing involves an activity (like driving) or a situation (like a restaurant) be sure you stick with it long enough for the anxiety to begin to come down. For example, if you really hate being "stuck" in a car, drive around the block 10–15 times. That way, you're always close to home (which makes it a lot less anxiety provoking) but you stick with it long enough for it to get boring. If even that feels too hard, just go sit in the car in the driveway for half an hour. This may feel a little ridiculous, but if it's the first step to getting you mobile and independent, it's totally worth doing it.

I had one patient who had had several traumatic experiences driving in situations in which her UC was not under good control and she ended up having to pull over to poop. In one instance she climbed into the back seat and pooped in a plastic shopping bag. In the other instance she pulled over on the side of the highway to poop in the bushes. When I started working with her, she hadn't driven herself anywhere in five years. Just getting into the driver's seat caused a rush of anxious arousal that was hard to tolerate. She stuck with it, though. The first time, she sat in the car with a good book and turned some music on. She just sat there until her anxiety went down, and then went back inside. The next time, she turned the car on and drove it up and down the driveway several times. Next, her husband drove her to a mall parking lot and she practiced driving there. (We had a good laugh about the fact that I had done the same thing that week with my 16-year-old daughter, who had recently gotten her learner's permit.) Eventually, she drove around the block near their home and finally drove to the supermarket, did the shopping and drove home. It took a long time to get there, but she was so pleased to have some adult independence back. (I also worked with that patient to reframe those previous experiences. I noted her resilience, resourcefulness and courage and pointed out that in the end she survived both situations and managed them pretty effectively. That reframe helped, too.)

I *don't* want you to pick something too hard. It's important to stick with whatever you choose until the anxiety begins to come down. If you abandon ship while the anxiety is still up or, worse yet, still rising, you might sensitize yourself. This shouldn't be a big scary thing. Just something small that you can imagine doing with some discomfort but can certainly imagine tolerating. (Sensitization isn't the end of the world – it can be fixed by going lower on the hierarchy and starting over. So don't sweat this too much.)

For example, if getting on a commuter train (the kind with no bathrooms aboard) feels too scary, just go to the train station and hang out for an hour. This may sound utterly ridiculous to you, but you're teaching your brain to stop associating riding trains with heightened anxiety, fear and danger. The next time you go, stand around on the platform for an hour, but don't board a train. Sit on a bench. Watch people come and go. Familiarize yourself with the rhythms of the station. This will get boring pretty quickly. The next time you go, board a train, go one stop, and then get off again. Wait for the next train going back toward home, board it, and go back home. Depending on the time of day, this may take a while, and you'll probably be pretty bored by the time you get home. That's good! Boredom is sort of like the opposite of fear. The *next* time you go, plan to ride the train for two or three stops. If you're feeling just fine, go all the way to some final destination that interests you. Then turn around and come home. The point is to realize that *any* task or situation that you have typically avoided and that feels challenging or anxiety provoking can be broken up into smaller pieces that feel quite doable.

If you typically avoid eating breakfast, you can start with a very small serving of a very safe food (say two little slices of banana). Do that on day one. The next day, try eating half of a banana. The day after that, you could try to eat a quarter cup of oatmeal with one or two banana slices. You get the idea. You start small, and see how the day goes. Chances are two slices of banana really aren't going to affect you that much one way or the other. Notice that I'm not suggesting you have a heaping platter of fried eggs, bacon, wholewheat toast with butter, hash browns and a big glass of orange juice the morning of the day you have an important meeting at work! But if you've been avoiding eating all together, this is an important aspect of avoidance to target early on.

Note that you may experience some physical discomfort just as a result of the *anxiety* involved in trying something you normally avoid. You may be gassy or feel your gut cramping a bit, even if you're not in flare at all. What we're mostly focused on here is the anxiety that goes with those sensations, not the sensations themselves. That is, one of the things you must keep in mind is that many kinds of GI discomfort are annoying and uncomfortable, but not cata-strophic and life limiting. In other words, one of the things you may need to expose yourself to is GI discomfort itself! That may sound a little crazy to you. If you have an IBD, you're "exposed" to GI discomfort all the time, right? Remember the lessons of the last chapter however – sometimes people with gut problems get so anxious about the very idea of experiencing GI symptoms that it becomes this huge, life altering, scary thing in and of itself. That's why subtle avoidance is so tricky to deal with – it's all about avoiding the *perceived* terrible consequences of having GI symptoms.

Obviously, if your doctor has told you to avoid specific foods, don't use those foods in this exercise. Moreover, if a certain food *always* predictably upsets your gut, or gives you gas, don't eat it. If you are having an active flare, then you should absolutely follow your doctor's advice about limiting or avoiding foods that might be medically problematic (e.g. avoiding high residue foods like celery if you have a partial stricture). But if there are foods that you have been avoiding because you've heard or have read online that they are "danger" foods, it's probably a good idea to expose yourself to a little bit of the food and see what happens.

Even more importantly, if you have been avoiding food-related *situations* then it is very important to pick one that you might be able to do. This might mean accepting a dinner invitation to a friend's home, but offering to make it "potluck" so you know there is at least one dish you can eat. It might mean meeting a colleague or friend at a restaurant and ordering only seltzer while they enjoy a full meal. This might actually make you pretty anxious. It is, admittedly, a little "weird" to do that. You might have to explain why. Just make clear that although you have severe dietary restrictions for health reasons, it is important to you to enjoy the person's company. You will almost certainly find that your anxiety and discomfort habituate or go down over the course of the meal. To keep the wait staff from repeatedly asking you if you're *sure* they can't get you anything, let them know up front that you won't be eating. This may feel like it violates an unstated social contract and it may make you feel uncomfortable, but the more you put yourself in situations like this, the less uncomfortable they will be over time. (You can always supplement the tip your friend leaves so that the server still makes a reasonable income from the meal.)

If you feel a little panicky in restaurants about the possibility of having to use the public restroom to defecate, it's important to ask yourself *why*. There are several reasons people might give to this. First, you might be afraid that a single restroom might be occupied when you really need it. You might have to "hold it" until the person using the room is done. One option is to use the opposite sex rest room. If it's truly just a single room (one for each sex) you won't be bothering anyone else. The other option is to use your deep breathing to manage the cramps and remind yourself that while you are uncomfortable, you have practiced "holding it" at home for short periods and can manage it for a minute or two. Second, many people worry about defecating in public restrooms because they worry about leaving disgusting smells behind and other people "knowing" what they were doing in there. Third, sometimes people worry about occupying a single rest room for a lengthy period of time knowing that *other* people might be frustrated because they also have to go. You might also worry about your dining companion wondering what on earth is taking you so long. It's important to remember that all these issues feel magnified to you well beyond what other people actually notice. Finally, some people just don't like using public restrooms at all – they might feel contaminated to you or just plain dirty or yucky.

The point of exposure therapy should be to reduce your anxiety in specific situations or environments in which you would usually feel somewhat anxious. It's far more important to be able to *go* to a restaurant with friends than it is to try to force yourself to eat greasy French fries or drink coffee. Really, greasy French fries aren't good for *anyone!* If you are *afraid* of food, that very fear may be exacerbating your gut distress. Food is such an important topic for people with GI issues that I've devoted an entire chapter to it. If you're one of those people who restricts your diet a great deal and consistently avoids a wide array of foods because you believe they're "dangerous triggers," please read Chapter 8 and then think about some exposure exercises you might try to address these issues. But it's far more important to focus on exposing yourself to social and occupational opportunities that you may have been missing out on for fear of GI symptoms disrupting the experience.

Indeed, the most devastating forms of avoidance for people with IBDs tend to be work or social situations in which they are afraid their gut will act up and be embarrassing or highly inconvenient and annoying to others. For example, you might not worry that much about driving someplace by yourself, because you know you can always pull over and find a restroom if you really need one. But you may be *very* anxious about driving with friends or colleagues because you worry a lot about asking someone else to pull over to a gas station or convenience store. This gets back to the core theme of *shame* that many people with IBDs struggle with. You just don't want to have to admit that there's anything wrong, and you certainly don't want to have to tell people exactly *what's* wrong.

Overcoming this type of avoidance is going to require a combination of cognitive reframing, exposure and behavioral experiments. Even if people were understanding, you might not want their pity. You don't want to be seen as "disabled" and it may be agonizing for you to have to ask other people to accommodate your needs and limitations. You may also not want to inconvenience others. Most adults pride themselves on being independent and competent. Most people want to see themselves as self-sufficient, accommodating and generous and not as needy, selfish or dependent. Situations that challenge those impressions may be very anxiety provoking. It's important to reframe these interpretations. It's always helpful to think about how you would feel if someone *else* needed your understanding or asked you to accommodate some specific need of theirs. The vast majority of us would feel honored to be taken into the person's confidence, and would be more than happy to be accommodating. So, why deny your friends and colleagues that opportunity? Don't see yourself as needy and dependent. See yourself as courageous and honest and proactive. Then *be* courageous and tell your friend or colleague that you might need to stop to use restroom along the way.

Here's a great example of a situation an IBD patient would typically have avoided, but decided to take a chance on while completing this treatment. This woman's extended family was planning a large family reunion that was going to take place at a camping facility with cabins, tent sites and a central dining hall/rec room. To make it affordable, the clan was booking as few cabins as possible. That meant the IBD patient would be sharing a cabin (with one bathroom!) with her husband, her adult son, her teenage son, and her adult son's fiancée. She was quite worried about the impact on everyone else of her needing to "monopolize" the toilet in the morning for an extended period of time, perhaps leaving it quite stinky in her wake. She was especially anxious about her son's fiancée, who did not know about her GI issues. She wanted to make a positive impression on this young woman, and appearing "selfish" and "gross" did *not* fit the image she wanted to portray! Rather than skipping the reunion entirely (which she would have been tempted to do previously) or spending a fortune on a separate cabin (which they really couldn't afford) she decided to be frank with her son's fiancée. She told her, in a very straightforward way, that she had a chronic GI condition. She also offered to get up a bit earlier than everyone else to try to complete her morning bathroom rituals before other people needed the room. She also brought a lovely scented candle and matches for the bathroom. In the end, she was pleasantly surprised by how delightful the long weekend was. Her initial anxiety abated quite quickly. The fiancée was understanding and respectful, and sharing the cabin turned out to be much less problematic than she had anticipated. In fact, the fiancée told the son (who told his mom) that she was so touched by her thoughtfulness and her resilience in managing a health issue. My patient was so glad she had not given in to anxious avoidance and denied herself this wonderful reunion experience and the chance to get to know her future daughter-in-law better.

Your homework this week is to think of several things you normally avoid or prefer to avoid that you would really like, in principle, to be able to do, and then figure out a way to sneak up on them and start doing them. You may have to start small and build your way up slowly. Start at the bottom of the anxiety hierarchy you constructed earlier in the chapter. In the text box below, please write down the two things you're going to try to do this week. I'd also like you to record your predictions about what you think will happen. When you try each of the things, you'll need to record what actually happens, including how uncomfortable you got and how long it took for the discomfort or anxiety to come down again.

Exposure exercises I can try:	Predictions: How uncomfortable will I get? How long will it last?	Results: How uncomfortable did I get? How long did it last?

Troubleshooting

If you find that you're having difficulty even getting yourself to do this assignment, see if you can identify the thoughts behind your reluctance. What is the worst thing that could happen? Would it be truly catastrophic? Do you see the point in trying to stop avoiding things? Most people with GI issues resent the (perceived) need to avoid things. They just don't see the point in pushing themselves to do things that might make them uncomfortable. Hopefully you're at the point by now where you understand that telling people about your GI issues isn't the end of the world, that in the vast majority of cases the "worst case" scenario doesn't come to pass, and even it *does* it may not be as bad as you once feared. The point of exposure therapy is to help you *reclaim your life*. Especially if you have secondary IBS, it's really important that you give this a shot. Exposure therapy *works* and is a central part of every effective intervention for anxiety and the avoidance that often develops of things that make people feel anxious. So if you've been hesitant to try it, do yourself a favor. Pick something really small and easy to do and *give it a shot*. Think of this as a behavioral experiment. You may think exposure is pointless or won't work. But if you've never tried it, you really don't *know* that that's true. Literally *thousands* of scientific studies have proven the efficacy of exposure therapy in helping people conquer anxiety and avoidance. Many studies have applied exposure therapy *specifically* to IBS, and a few studies have even shown that it's highly effective at treating anxiety that is co-morbid or secondary to Crohn's and colitis. It works. You just have to prove it to yourself.

Mind you, lots of different kinds of things can happen when people first start trying exposure therapy. If you tried it, but had difficulty with the assignment, or you found that the anxiety did *not* come down, then you probably tried to do something too hard. The key to exposure therapy is to start small and *stick with it*. For example, suppose you decided to try to take the commuter train into town. You anticipated it would raise your SUD score to about 25. But when you got on the train, your SUD score shot up to 40 or 50, and you ended up getting off at the next stop. Next time, just go to the train station and hang out with a good book or magazine for an hour. Don't even get on a train! The idea is to sneak up on the things that make you anxious, and to do it in a way that lets you associate those things with feeling calm, relaxed and even bored, rather than anxious. Once being in the train station itself is just boring, then it may be time to get on a train. But *plan* to go only one stop. Then get off. Then get back on the next train and go one more stop. Then get off. Keep doing this until that gets boring. (It may also be time consuming, depending on the time of day and the train schedule.)

Another difficulty people have is that they don't stick with an activity long enough. Suppose you make yourself go to the supermarket or the home store to buy a few items and wait in line. You might "get through it" by going through the express line and getting out of there as fast as possible, but chances are your anxiety will still be up when you leave. The goal should be to go to the store and just hang out until you get bored. The first day, you might just sit in your car in the parking lot for an hour. I know this may sound absurd, but remember that we want to set you up for success. You want to pick something to do that is predictably boring and doable and that won't arouse too much distress. The next day you might walk around the store for a half hour at a fairly empty time of day without even buying anything. (Put a basket over your arm and read a lot of labels so you don't feel goofy.) The point is to stick with it until your anxiety begins to come down.

Often, people have the opposite "problem" with exposure therapy – the first thing they try doesn't make them anxious *enough*! It ends up being much easier and less anxiety provoking or uncomfortable than they predicted. That's actually a fine way to start. Just be sure that you progress to the next thing up on the hierarchy. Exposure therapy only helps if you are tackling things that are at least a little bit anxiety provoking.

The other thing to remember about exposure therapy is that it isn't a one-shot cure. You have to keep doing it, slowly working your way up your anxiety hierarchy. I usually suggest that people practice something on their list *every day* or at least every other day. You can do the same thing a few days in a row. Ask to use a bathroom at a different retail establishment every day for several days in a row. You should find that you don't get as anxious the second day as you did the first day, and the anxiety should come down even faster. After a few days, you should try the next thing up on your list.

It's also important to target any types of subtle avoidance you engage in. Ironically, things that may be perfectly reasonable and adaptive coping strategies when you are in an active flare may turn into maladaptive subtle avoidance when you are in remission. This is especially true if you have developed secondary IBS. For example, if you're having an active flare, it's perfectly reasonable to carry emergency supplies with you when you are out and about, including a change of underwear, a pack of wet wipes and some anti-diarrheal medication. This is quite sensible, especially if you are actually experiencing fecal incontinence from time to time. You will be much better off if you *go out* and live your life (emergency pack in tow) than if you stay home for fear of incontinence and avoid work, love and play. But when you're *no longer in flare* it's probably a good idea to start leaving that emergency bag at home. Carrying it around all the time for *fear* that your gut will act up may actually exacerbate the underlying fear, even if it makes you feel more secure in the moment.

Lots of times people who engage in subtle avoidance don't even end up "needing" whatever they're carrying or doing. That is, you may scope out the locations of bathrooms, and then most of the time find you do not need them. Sometimes people say they just feel "more secure" if they have their anti-anxiety medication with them. Just carrying that Xanax in your pocket makes you more relaxed. Ironically, trying to stop subtle avoidance behaviors is sometimes the most difficult thing to convince yourself to do. Please note that these exercises do *not* apply to medications that have been prescribed by your doctor to target the underlying disease process and manage symptoms during active flares. *ALWAYS* follow your doctor's medical advice when it comes to treatment for IBD. What I am talking about here are the *extra* things you might be doing to avoid the very *possibility* of experiencing GI sensations or finding yourself in an awkward or uncomfortable or embarrassing situation, or just feeling anxious, especially when your IBD is in remission.

The reason to eat breakfast, to leave the benzo at home, to forego that morning dose of "just-in-case" Imodium or to sit in the middle of the aisle is that these things are all part of a pattern of thoughts and behaviors that keeps your gut in control of your life. Every time you check that the Lomotil or the Bentyl is in your purse or briefcase or glove compartment, you give a bit more ground to letting your gut control your life. "Gut distress and anxiety are intolerable and must be avoided at all costs" is the message you send your brain. So eat a small breakfast. Try not taking the Imodium. Go ahead and sit in the middle of row. Go to the mall without immediately scoping out where the nearest restroom is. Tell your co-worker in the next cubicle, in a matter-of-fact way, why you have to visit the restroom so often. By sending your brain the message that you can do these things "safely" you help reduce the sense of "danger" people with gut problems often experience. *You* have the power to turn your GI problems from an ever-present, disabling, shameful condition to an annoying inconvenience that doesn't really impact your quality of life all that much. And that's what this program is all about.

8 Diet

One of the biggest myths about GI disorders is that there is an ideal diet that will reduce or resolve symptoms for most or all people. IBD patients almost always ask their doctors for recommendations about food and diet as a way to control their symptoms and improve or even cure their disease, and you'd think there would be sensible, evidence-based advice that doctors could give. Unfortunately, there is much less scientific or medical evidence regarding the impact of diet on IBD than you would hope, which is kind of bizarre when you think about it. So your doctor may well not have much to say that's actually all that helpful. This makes many IBD patients turn to the internet, to support groups and chat rooms to try to figure out what has "worked" for other people. The situation gets even more confusing when you have secondary IBS. There is a *ton* of advice out there about diet and IBS, and the advice for IBD patients is often parallel to or overlapping the advice for IBS patients. You will see all kinds of recommendations, in books, on the web, and even in the research literature. Eat a high fiber diet. Eat a low-fiber diet. Eat only the right kind of fiber. Avoid all milk products with lactose and switch to soy products instead. Avoid soy products at all costs. Eat *some* legumes but not others. Avoid all legumes. Avoid wheat and gluten. Avoid *all* grains. Avoid all sugars. Avoid eggs. Avoid meat and eat a vegetarian or even vegan diet. Eat a Paleolithic diet low in carbs and *high* in meat. Avoid raw vegetables, beans and fruit. Eat lots of vegetables. Eat a very low carbohydrate (low FODMAP) diet. Avoid spicy food. Avoid greasy food. Avoid fat altogether. Take probiotics or mint or ginger. Don't take probiotics or mint or ginger. If you tried to follow *all* the advice out there about "trigger" foods, you'd end up with nothing at all on your plate except a pile of plain white rice. Not a very appetizing, nutritious or practical solution.

So it would be really nice if there were clear cut, scientifically sound recommendations about how to manage diet to minimize inflammation and IBD symptoms. Unfortunately, we're just not there yet. We do know that a traditional "Western" diet, high in processed food, sugar and saturated fat and low in fiber, whole grains and vegetables, has terrible effects on the intestinal microbiome and is associated with greater risk for IBD. We also know that dietary changes can impact the diversity of the microbiome and immune system

DOI: 10.4324/9781003057635-9

reactivity, and *may* turn out to be an important adjunctive therapy for people with IBDs. Sadly, doing the kind of research necessary to establish the efficacy and the mechanisms of change in specific diets is really hard.[1] You need a *lot* of people who are willing to eat controlled diets and log everything they put into their mouth for a long time. They also need to be willing to give blood and poop samples so the researchers can actually track the impact of the dietary intervention on inflammation and the microbiome. Although we're learning more every day, we still don't really know enough to make specific, targeted recommendations that will work for everyone.[2] That leaves most folks with IBDs to turn to nonmedical resources (like the internet) for advice. Unfortunately, most of the patient-targeted dietary recommendations on the internet focus on *restricting* foods or food groups and are highly conflicting and inconsistent. This is particularly concerning because people with IBDs often suffer from nutrient malabsorption, so eliminating whole classes of foods often makes malnutrition and nutrient deficiencies *worse*. [3] The biggest concern for people with IBDs should be *getting sufficient nutrition*. This means that IBD patients should follow the least restrictive diet possible. If you do end up "cutting" a food or food group, you may need to add in supplements or food substitutes to ensure that you're getting sufficient calories, vitamins, minerals, proteins, fats and carbohydrates, *all* of which are necessary for life, health and vitality.

Even if you want to eat a varied diet in principle, another problem is that people with IBDs often develop *fear of food* and are at heightened risk of developing avoidant restrictive food intake disorder (ARFID). ARFID is a new diagnostic category that captures several kinds of problematic food avoidance. In all cases, the avoidance of food leads to problems of some kind, which can include weight loss, malnutrition or even just significant social impairment. IBD patients who also develop ARFID are at particular risk of malnutrition.[4] Why would IBD patients develop fear of food and start avoiding lots of different foods? Simple. People are afraid of experiencing pain, diarrhea and life disruptions if they eat the wrong thing, or eat it at the wrong time. The Fear of Food Questionnaire (FFQ) in the Appendix will give you a good idea if this is true of you. Note that fear of food (and ARFID) are totally different from eating disorders like anorexia and bulimia nervosa. People with ARFID aren't afraid of gaining weight and don't typically have distorted beliefs about being "fatter" than they are. To the contrary, they are often distressed by the weight loss, nutritional deficiencies and interference with normal socializing and functioning that come with avoiding lots of different foods.

Some ARFID patients were super picky eaters as kids and remain super picky eaters as adults, to the extent that their limited diet compromises nutrition and caloric intake. Those folks aren't afraid of food, they just really hate most foods. The textures or smells or tastes of lots of different foods not only aren't appealing, they're actively disgusting to them. An example would be folks who are very sensitive to sulfur compounds found in eggs and cruciferous vegetables like broccoli. Imagine trying to eat something that smelled to you like rotten farts. Not very appealing. In fact, some of these folks view lots of foods as inedible non-food substances that they have no idea how to eat, sort of like if someone told you to eat a plastic bag or a brick. It's not just that you wouldn't want to. It's that you wouldn't even know how. Treatment for picky eating ARFID in adults generally involves some cognitive reframing and a lot of practice and graded exposure to foods that aren't appealing, but aren't actively disgusting.

Chemical sensitivity to the smell and taste of food can work the other way too. Artichokes have a compound in them that some people can taste and other people can't. If you are sensitive to it, artichokes have an exquisite taste – sort of a hollow, sweet, aluminum taste that fills your whole mouth and palate. It's hard to describe, but it's incredibly delicious. But if you *can't* taste it, artichokes will seem like a lot of effort to get a tiny bit of pointless, tasteless mush. This isn't a moral issue or a question of maturity or the willingness to try new things. It's a fluke of genetics. You're either born with the ability to taste/smell that chemical or you're not. If you are a picky eater because you just don't enjoy the taste or smell or texture of some foods, but you still eat a varied and balanced diet, don't worry about it, you don't have ARFID. And don't let people bully you or tease you about your preferences.

The *other* group of folks with ARFID, however, are people who might like the food itself, but are terribly afraid of experiencing something awful during or after eating the food. Examples include fear of choking on the food, fear of feeling nauseous or throwing up after eating the food, or fear of developing painful GI symptoms like gas, cramping or urgent diarrhea after eating the food. Most folks with IBD who go on to develop ARFID are in this category. You may *wish* you could eat certain foods, and may miss them, but you're so afraid of triggering painful or debilitating GI symptoms that you avoid lots of different foods and whole food groups to try to stave off those aversive consequences. While it is natural to want to limit your discomfort and diarrhea, it's also important not to get into the habit of avoiding or restricting your diet too much.

Treatment for fear-based ARFID is all about graded exposure – trying small amounts of feared foods one at a time and tolerating the *anxiety* eating the food causes until it goes away or habituates. The vast majority of the time, nothing else terrible happens. It's just that eating the food makes you anxious because you're *expecting* something awful to happen. Of course, as you know, anxiety can cause GI symptoms all by itself. So chances are, it wasn't (just) the food that made you feel bad to begin with. And if you've developed visceral hypersensitivity, then part of the goal is to learn to tolerate some GI sensations and remind yourself that while they may be uncomfortable, they're not dangerous and they may actually be quite normal. Everyone produces gas. It's a natural by-product of digestion. Some foods tend to create more gas than others. That's normal. The goal here is to learn not to get overly focused on the sensations of gas and bloating, so that you don't have to be *afraid* of eating foods that naturally create gas as result of fermentation and digestion. As you stop catastrophizing and being upset and angry about those sensations, you will actually start to *notice* them less and they will become less uncomfortable and less bothersome.

So the overarching goal should be to eat as varied, nutrient dense a diet as possible, rich in whole natural foods from lots of different categories to maintain nutrition, weight, a diverse microbiome and health. That does not mean, however, that dietary changes can't help. Dietary changes can sometimes be *useful* in helping you minimize some of the *discomfort* associated with GI symptoms. And moving away from an impoverished, processed food Western diet may well reduce inflammation and contribute to longer term health and even remission. There are some basic principles that are usually helpful for most people to understand and incorporate into their dietary choices. There are also some specific food choices that *many* (but not all!) people with GI problems can benefit from. Below, we detail some of the most common recommendations out there and why they might or might not make sense for you.

Please note that all of the diet advice in this chapter (and the references to the scientific literature) applies to IBD patients when you are *not* having an active flare. However, there are certain dietary changes your doctor will advise you to make during active flares, and you should, of course, follow your doctor's advice. In particular, your doctor may recommend a "low-residue diet" in which fiber (particularly insoluble fiber) and other foods that are harder for your body to digest are restricted. This is particularly important if you have been diagnosed with intestinal strictures, in which part of the intestinal wall becomes thickened by scar tissue and the tube through which food must pass becomes too narrow and rigid. If you eat too much fiber, chunky food like nuts or popcorn, or stringy food like celery, it can actually cause a blockage at the point of the stricture. Note, however, that doctors typically recommend a low-residue/low-fiber diet for *short-term use* during disease flare ups or following surgery to help with recovery. It is *not* a general eating plan for all people with IBD all the time.

Fiber

Few dietary recommendations get people with GI problems more agitated than the simplistic recommendation to "eat more fiber." A high fiber diet generally reduces the risk of developing an IBD. Doctors sometimes recommend increasing dietary fiber by adding wheat bran (usually in the form of cereal) or taking Metamucil (psyllium) or Citrucel (methylcellulose). One study found that daily doses of psyllium were as effective as mesalamine in maintaining remission in UC.[5] But lots of folks with IBD will find that adding "fiber" makes their symptoms worse, and sometimes your doctor will explicitly tell you to *limit* fiber (by eating a low-residue diet) to "rest" your intestines or help you recover post-surgically.

One of the reasons for these confusing findings and conflicting advice is that there are two different *kinds* of dietary fiber. Neither kind is fully "digested" by the acids, enzymes and symbiotic bacteria in our bodies, but they act very differently as they pass through our digestive system.

Insoluble fiber is the kind of fiber found in the bran of whole grains, leafy green vegetables (like lettuce and spinach) and fruit and vegetable *skins*.

Insoluble fiber does not dissolve in water and passes through your digestive system largely intact. In fact, sometimes you can still recognize the food perfectly well when it comes out the other end. (For example, whole corn kernels, shreds of lettuce or spinach or bits of tomato skin may be easy to identify in very loose stools.) In general, insoluble fiber adds *bulk* to stool. All in all, this generally makes stools larger and softer, as long as you drink plenty of water. It also decreases "transit time" through the colon. That is, the more insoluble fiber you eat, the faster your stools will move through you. If you are *currently* suffering primarily from constipation (which is unusual, but not unheard of for folks with an IBD, especially if they have developed secondary IBS), adding a bit more insoluble fiber to your diet is probably a good idea. Just remember to drink more water too! In general, diets relatively high in insoluble fiber promote regular bowel movements and prevent constipation. Insoluble fiber also helps your body move toxic waste through your colon in less time. This may be part of the reason that high fiber diets are linked to a lower incidence of certain cancers.

But! Relatively few people with an IBD develop constipation predominant secondary IBS. For *most* people with an underlying IBD, foods high in insoluble fiber should be eaten only in moderation, and limited even more strictly during active flares or if you have significant strictures. The *last* thing you need is looser, more watery stools that pass through the colon more quickly. That doesn't mean you should avoid these foods altogether. Whole grains and leafy green vegetables are an important part of a healthy diet. It does mean that they should probably be eaten in small quantities at a time, combined with other foods that will cushion their effect. *While in flare*, you should probably focus more on refined grains with *less* insoluble fiber. This means avoiding whole wheat bread or cornmeal tortillas in favor of sourdough and French breads, and eating more oats and white rice. You should probably also *peel* any fruit or vegetable that has a tough skin, including apples, tomatoes and eggplants, and try not to eat hard seeds like those found in tomatoes or poppy or sesame seeds. If you love salad, eat baby or micro greens or butter lettuce, not mature iceberg or romaine lettuce. Love spinach? Buy baby spinach and cut off the stems before steaming or cooking it down in the microwave with a bit of olive oil. In other words, find ways to incorporate these healthful whole foods into your diet in ways that don't risk worsening diarrhea or causing an obstruction.

Soluble fiber does dissolve in water. It's found in bananas, carrots, oats and oat bran, rice, the flesh (but not the skins) of potatoes and sweet potatoes and the flesh (but not the skins or seeds) of many other fruits and vegetables including apples, avocado, berries, tomatoes, beets, eggplant, squash and pumpkin, and in nuts, beans and peas. While soluble fiber is not completely digested, it does break down into a gel-like substance as it passes through your digestive tract. Thus, soluble fiber tends to make your stools softer, but also helps them adhere and gives them shape. Soluble fiber also enhances intestinal mucus. That may sound gross, but it's a good thing. Even more importantly, soluble fiber is partially fermented by colonic bacteria, which produce short-chain fatty acids (SCFAs). SCFAs modulate the immune response of different cell types in the intestines and reduce inflammation. They also help shift the balance of species of gut microbes toward more beneficial species.[6] Indeed, one study which focused on reducing processed carbohydrates, but increasing consumption of whole, natural foods high in soluble fiber led to significant reduction in IBD symptoms.[7] Overall, consuming enough soluble fiber is actually important for long-term health and remission in IBD patients.[8]

The best solution for most people is to combine soluble and *small* amounts of insoluble fiber at every meal. For example, instead of having raisin bran for breakfast (where almost all the fiber is insoluble), have a bowl of oatmeal (soluble) with strawberries (soluble) and blueberries (a bit of insoluble in the skin). Or better yet, make your own granola bars with whole rolled oats (soluble) and a smooth nut butter (some soluble and some insoluble) and have it with a banana. This is a high protein, deliciously satisfying breakfast that provides lots of heart healthy omega-3 fats, vitamins and minerals and should help calm a crampy gut and reduce diarrhea.

If you want to increase your consumption of soluble fiber quickly and easily, psyllium seeds may be a good source for you. Psyllium, also known as plantago or isphagula, contains very high levels of soluble fiber. The husk or coat of the psyllium seed is about 30% mucilage – exactly the stuff that turns into slippery, soft, water absorbing soluble fiber in the gut. It acts as a soothing lubricant and helps absorb excess water, making it a useful intervention for both constipation and diarrhea. (This was the type of fiber used in the study that helped bring UC patients into remission.) Note that psyllium is the main ingredient in Metamucil. So if Metamucil aggravates your symptoms, psyllium is unlikely to be helpful.

Milk Products

Many people with gut problems believe that avoiding milk products can be a good idea. This is based on the assumption that lactose (the sugar in milk) is "difficult to digest" for many people. If your GI symptoms are really caused in part by lactose intolerance, then eliminating milk products that are high in lactose is a really good idea.

There is some evidence that individuals with Crohn's Disease are at heightened risk for lactose intolerance.[9] The hydrogen and/or methane breath tests described in Chapter 1 do a pretty good job of identifying lactose intolerance in people with IBDs, so if you're pretty sure your symptoms get worse after consuming dairy products, it's worth having it done. However, a large review study concluded that lactose maldigestion in IBD was dependent on ethnic makeup of the population (just like lactose intolerance for everyone else) and *not* on disease itself. Moreover, consumption of dairy foods may actually *decrease* the risk of IBD.[10] If you're not actually lactose intolerant, there is really *no need* to eliminate dairy products from your diet. They are a wonderful source of complete protein, calcium, and vitamin D, all of which can be tough to get enough of when you have an IBD. In addition, GI patients who avoid dairy are much more likely to show reduced bone density. If you don't like milk, eat yogurt or aged cheeses or try kefir. Yogurt and kefir are both probiotic foods with active bacterial cultures that can help re-populate your microbiome and contain relatively little lactose (because the active cultures have already fermented it). If you are lactose intolerant, try Lactaid products and keep getting all the calcium and vitamin D you need for your bones.

Wheat and Gluten

The story with wheat and other gluten containing products is very similar to the story with milk products. Some people with GI problems swear that eliminating gluten was the magic bullet they were looking for. But most people find that eliminating gluten does them no good whatsoever. Why? Probably because the people who benefited from eliminating gluten *really* had undiagnosed Celiac Disease.

It is true that individuals with inflammatory bowel disease are at elevated risk for *also* having Celiac Disease (and vice versa) relative to the general population.[11] After all, both are autoimmune disorders. If you *do* have Celiac, then you absolutely should eliminate gluten. However, assuming that your early diagnostic work-ups eliminated Celiac Disease as a contributing factor to your GI distress, there is really no need to eliminate gluten from your diet. "Gluten-free" diets are a fad at the moment, and it is lovely for people with Celiac Disease that so many gluten-free products and foods are now available at both restaurants and grocery stores. But if you don't have Celiac Disease, it's almost certainly not worth the expense and the trouble. In addition, eliminating gluten means eliminating whole classes of foods (especially anything containing wheat) and, as we know, the more varied your diet is the more likely you are to get adequate nutrition.

Probiotics

Probiotics refer to live microorganisms (like bacteria) that can be ingested either in food (as in yogurt) or in a supplement pill form that are helpful to overall health. The microorganisms survive inside the person who eats them, join the existing microflora in the gut and contribute to the health of the person. Remember, our digestive system depends on millions of bacteria that *normally* inhabit our gut and help us digest our food. Probiotics are a way of supplementing that ecosystem with more helpful bacteria. Without those critters to help us break down food, it passes through relatively undigested, resulting in diarrhea. In fact, one of the most important functions of these microflora are that they ferment undigested carbohydrates and soluble fiber in the colon – thus playing a crucial role in creating the helpful, gel-like substance that binds stool, but keeps it soft. There is growing evidence that consuming probiotics can be helpful to people with UC in particular, although the evidence for folks with Crohn's Disease is less clear.[12] As with any nutritional product, people with an IBD should consult with their doctors before using a probiotic supplement. It may not be a good idea during active flare ups, but may be quite helpful at other times, particularly for maintaining remission in UC.

The easiest way to consume probiotics is to eat or drink dairy products (like yogurt, buttermilk and kefir) in which the "active, live cultures" are exactly the probiotic bacteria we want in our guts. (Such combinations are natural "synbiotics" which contain both a helpful bacterial probiotic and a nourishing pre-biotic, a food that helps keep the bacteria alive.) Consuming probiotics in dairy products is easy, and there's some evidence that the milk product itself buffers the cultures, keeps them alive while in storage, and helps them survive the harrowing trip through the stomach acids to arrive in the gut alive and well. Even mildly lactose intolerant people often find that they can eat yogurt without any ill effects, since the bacteria in the cultures have already broken down a good deal of the lactose.

The alternative is to purchase a probiotic supplement, usually in a pill or tablet form. Be sure to get one that has an enteric coating. Otherwise the cultures are unlikely to survive exposure to stomach acid. Remember that "supplements" that are sold over the counter are not regulated by the Food and Drug Administration and many products don't really contain what they claim on the label. Talk to your doctor about which formulation and brand might be best for you to try.[13]

Peppermint

Mint has been used for millennia as a soothing digestive aid. It turns out that peppermint oil actually *does* relax the smooth muscles of the intestinal tract, can reduce visceral sensitivity, and may have some anti-inflammatory activity as well.[14] This makes it helpful for folks with secondary IBS.[15] There just isn't much data available yet on whether mint is helpful for folks with an IBD, but it does seem to be safe, and there are a few possible mechanisms by which it might be helpful.[16] If you want to try peppermint oil, it's best to buy it in the form of enteric coated capsules (such as IBgard). This is important, because straight peppermint oil hitting the stomach can cause reflux and belching that is quite unpleasant and tastes surprisingly *terrible*, not minty fresh. There are no controlled studies of the use of menthol or peppermint in IBDs, but if your doctor approves it, there is no harm in trying it.

Ginger

Ginger, like mint, has been used for millennia as a digestive aid, particularly for the treatment of nausea and vomiting. There is data to suggest that ginger (taken fresh, drunk as tea, used as a spice in food or taken as a supplement) may indeed reduce *gastric* (or stomach) distress, nausea and vomiting. However, since both IBD (and secondary IBS) typically affect the intestines, *not* the stomach, ginger is unlikely to provide substantial relief to most people. However, it is

possible that ginger may have some useful anti-inflammatory effects in the gut
For example, there is one study (in rats) suggesting that ginger extract may
exert some anti-inflammatory properties in animal models of ulcerative colitis.[17] There is one clinical trial currently underway in humans testing the
impact of ginger (versus a placebo) on inflammatory markers in UC.[18] So the
bottom line is that we just don't know yet if ginger is helpful. However, if you
like the taste, there is certainly no harm in adding ginger to your diet, and it
might prove helpful.

Gassy Foods

Many people with IBDs and especially with secondary IBS complain of gas and
flatulence. Some foods are definitely more likely to cause gas than others.
Legumes (including beans, lentils and soy), cruciferous vegetables (including
cabbage, broccoli, cauliflower, and Brussels sprouts) and onions all contain compounds that lead to the production of gas in the digestive tract as they are broken
down. There are no well controlled scientific studies of the impact of eliminating
or reducing gas producing foods on IBD. There are simple steps that can be
taken to reduce the gassy by-products of some of these foods, however. Over the
counter supplements such as Beano and Bean-zyme contain an enzyme (alpha-
galactosidase) that helps break down the gas causing compounds in legumes and
cruciferous vegetables before they reach the large intestine. There *are* scientific
studies supporting the efficacy of these enzyme supplements at reducing gas and
flatulence in people without any GI disorder.[19] So if excessive, bothersome gas,
bloating or flatulence typically follows consumption of these foods for you, it's
certainly worth giving Beano or a similar product a try.

Soy Products

As noted above, soy beans are legumes (just like black beans, kidney beans,
cannellini beans, chickpeas and lentils) and belong to the class of foods that can
cause excess intestinal gas (and diarrhea) in some people. This is one of the
main reasons that switching from cow's milk to soy milk products may do you
no good at all, and may actually make your symptoms worse. If you are actually lactose intolerant, or if you just really like tofu, edamame, or soy milk and
want to be able to eat soy products with no difficulty, products like Beano may
help. Don't expect soy products to be the silver bullet that cures your GI
symptom. But don't view soy as "dangerous" either. It is neither. In moderation, like just about any other food, soy products can be part of a nutritious
balanced diet for just about everyone. Like milk products, they are high in
protein (though it's not complete and needs to be supplemented with a grain
like rice or wheat) and calcium. Miso, which is a fermented paste made from
soy and (often) a grain, salt and a type of mold spore, is a great probiotic food
that adds a delicious umami taste to many dishes and is often used in traditional
Japanese cooking.

Fructose

Fructose is a naturally occurring sugar that is found many fruits and quite a few vegetables. Some people with GI problems swear that fructose makes their symptoms worse, and that avoiding fruit (especially apples, pears, melons, peaches and cherries) and other sources of fructose (like the infamous high fructose corn syrup) helps enormously. When these sugar molecules are not absorbed in the small intestine, they pass on to the large intestine, where they will be fermented by bacteria. This can lead to excess gas, a change in intestinal motility and discomfort or even diarrhea. There is some evidence that people with Crohn's Disease (but not ulcerative colitis) may show higher rates of fructose malabsorption than healthy controls.[20] It would be extremely difficult, impractical and probably unwise, however, to eliminate all of these natural foods from your diet. By all means, cut out soda and other highly processed, nutritionally empty foods that are flavored with high fructose corn syrup. But eliminating natural fruits like apples, melons, cherries and pears will deprive you of vitamins, minerals, and a wonderful source of soluble fiber.

Sorbitol, Xylitol and Low-Calorie "Fake" Sugars

Sorbitol and Xylitol are considered sugar "substitutes" because, although they taste very sweet, they are generally not digested or absorbed very well, so they are lower calorie and don't cause blood glucose levels to spike the way other sugars do. They both occur naturally in some foods, (especially fruits) but are often uses as additives in a variety of diet and "sugar free" processed foods, including baked goods, candy and gum. There is no question that these food additives can increase gas, bloating and diarrhea as they are broken down by bacteria in the large intestine. While I don't generally recommend avoiding foods, these low-calorie sugar substitutes don't really count as "food" because they have almost no nutritional value whatsoever.

Truly fake sugars (such as saccharine, aspartame and sucralose) are even worse for you, and should be avoided by people with an IBD. There is increasing evidence that these synthetic chemicals have terrible effects on the microbiome and probably aren't helpful for weight loss anyway, since they contribute to insulin resistance.[21] In general, eating fake food is a really bad idea. If you see a fake or manufactured sugar on the label of a processed food, put it back on the shelf, head back to the produce section, and buy yourself some beautiful fresh fruit instead.

Coffee

Coffee – even decaffeinated coffee – stimulates intestinal motility in almost everyone.[22] Many people with GI disorders choose to avoid coffee (and other caffeinated beverages such as black tea and soda) in the hopes that it will reduce intestinal distress. There have been no good scientific studies of the impact of coffee or caffeine on IBD (or IBS for that matter). Lots of people with an IBD *believe* that drinking coffee might make their GI symptoms worse, but mostly they drink it anyway.[23] There is a little bit of evidence that drinking coffee may actually increase beneficial bacteria in the gut.[24] On the other hand, eliminating these beverages from your diet is relatively easy to do, and there may be health benefits beyond GI symptoms. Most people find that they sleep better and enjoy more sustained energy during the day when they wean themselves off caffeine. A cup of mint or ginger tea can be a pleasant way to start the day, if you crave that morning cup. On the other hand, since there is very little data suggesting that coffee exacerbates GI symptoms, it's unlikely to be the real culprit. If you're really curious, try eliminating coffee for a week or two (be prepared for some headaches the first few days if you're a real addict). See if your GI symptoms improve. Then reintroduce coffee and see what happens. But be careful not to catastrophize the outcome! Say you drink half a cup of coffee in the morning and 15 minutes later you find that you experience a strong urge to defecate. Is this really so bad? Hot liquid hitting the stomach in the morning stimulates intestinal activity for *most* people. That could actually be a good thing! After all, many people with an IBD would like to know that their bodies are predictable. You have to defecate sometime during the day. Why not first thing in the morning, halfway through your cup of coffee, but before you take your shower? On the other hand, if coffee truly makes you feel ill, then by all means, avoid it.

Meat and Eggs

Red meat, dark meat from poultry, poultry skin, pork and egg yolks are commonly perceived as dangerous "trigger" foods and are listed on many IBD and IBS related websites as foods to avoid at all costs. *There is no data from any study suggesting that this is true.* You may choose to avoid different types of meat for any of a number of reasons, including on religious, environmental, ecological, economic or moral grounds. There are certainly dozens of well-designed studies suggesting that diets *relatively* low in red meat and saturated fat contribute to an overall healthy lifestyle, and reduce your long-term risk of heart disease and some cancers. There is also evidence that a diet that is too heavy in meat and saturated fat and too low in fiber, fruits and vegetables increases the life time risk of developing an IBD[25] and is associated with worse disease course in folks who have an IBD.[26] But none of that means you shouldn't eat meat at all.

The main problems with meat in America are two-fold. First, we tend to eat too much of it in a single "serving" and probably have it too often. Second, too many of the animals we eat are raised in inhumane ways and fed unnatural diets. For example, most cows are fed on grain (as opposed to grass) because it's cheaper. Eating grain (especially corn) is really bad for cows because their digestive system evolved over hundreds of thousands of years to digest *grass*. Corn causes them all sorts of digestive problems, including ulcers and infections, and leads directly to the overuse of antibiotics on feedlots. Ironically, it is these animals that suffer from horrible gastrointestinal problems, and their fat is probably far worse for our cardiovascular health than the fat of grass fed, organically raised animals, because the ratio of omega 6 to omega 3 is thrown out of whack. Similarly, chickens raised in crowded factory farms have truly awful living conditions and are fed mostly grains and animal by-products. They are also dosed constantly with low level antibiotics, which helps give rise to resistant strains of salmonella.

Egg yolks have been demonized by a number of different groups, especially because they contain high levels of cholesterol. They are also typically listed in the "must avoid" column on many lists of GI trigger foods because of their high fat content. But egg yolks *also* contain high levels of vitamins E, A and D, folate, riboflavin and good omega fatty acids, all of which are essential and contribute substantially to health in many ways. If you throw out the yolk, you throw out most of the nutritional value in an egg beyond the pure protein, and this is a terrible idea for someone with an IBD who might be having difficulty getting adequate nutrition. So *don't* throw out those yolks! Eat whole eggs, as nature intended.

So if you're going to eat meat and eggs, do so moderately and responsibly. If you care about animal welfare, eat meat less often, but pay more to buy organic, grass fed, pasture raised, free range meat and eggs raised in humane ways. Organic eggs laid by pastured hens tend to contain even more of the good fats and vitamins we need, and you can feel good about supporting ethical and ecologically sound farming practices. Remember how DDT almost caused the extinction of eagles because their eggshells got so thin they broke when the mother tried to sit on them? Organic chicken eggs have *much* harder shells than non-organic eggs. Think about it. A pound of organic grass feed beef or a dozen organic, pastured hen eggs costs more than twice as much as the cheap inhumane factory food alternative, but it's better for the animals and the environment *and* it's better for you.

Fried Food and Fatty Food

Eating a diet with very limited fried food is probably a good idea for everyone. A huge platter of barbecued spareribs or fried chicken, French fries or greasy biscuits and coleslaw or corn-on-the-cob slathered in butter may or may not send you running to the bathroom, but it won't be good for you, no matter how you look at it. Eat fried and fatty foods occasionally and in small portions to save your waistline and your heart. This is good dietary advice for all of us.

Spicy Foods

"Spice" can refer to any number of substances that are used to flavor food, making it more pungent, aromatic or tastier. Cinnamon and nutmeg are both "spices" that do not seem to contribute to GI symptoms at all. Some of the ingredients in curry – the classic Indian combination used to spice many foods –

include ginger and turmeric, which may actually reduce gastrointestinal distress for some people. Capsaicin, which is the chemical that makes chili peppers "hot," may in fact contribute somewhat to abdominal pain in individuals with secondary IBS. One study[27] did find evidence in people with IBS of increased sensitivity and density in the sigmoid colon of nerves that respond to capsaicin. In addition, the density of those nerve cells was correlated or related to abdominal pain in individuals with IBS. On the other hand, capsaicin actually has anti-inflammatory properties, and could be potentially helpful reducing intestinal inflammation.[28] So there is a chance that reducing or avoiding exposure to "hot" or "picante" foods might be helpful. You yourself can be the best judge. As with coffee, it might be worth doing a behavioral experiment – avoiding those foods for several weeks, and then intentionally eating a spicy meal to see what happens. As always, the key is to avoid catastrophizing the results of eating those foods. You may be a bit uncomfortable, which is annoying. But it does *not* need to be a catastrophe.

Low FODMAP Diet

The low FODMAP diet is one of the most restrictive diets out there, and there is some evidence that it is helpful (in the short term) for secondary IBS in patients with IBD in remission who are still experiencing GI symptoms. FODMAP stands for "Fermentable Oligo-, Di- and Mono-saccharides and Polyols." These are all carbohydrates that are broken down, or *fermented* by the intestinal microbiome – those symbiotic bacteria that live in the gut. In fact, these are all the *pre-biotic* foods that nourish our microbiome. High FODMAP foods *do* reliably cause more gas and water content in the gut as a by-product of the fermentation process. They do this equally for everyone. However, this is only problematic in the context of visceral hypersensitivity, and only IBS patients (and some patients with inflammatory bowel disease and secondary IBS) are particularly bothered by it.

The diet attempts to eliminate all the carbohydrates which are broken down into sugars during digestion and may exacerbate gas, flatulence, cramping and diarrhea. It's really a combination of lots of other advice – and includes eliminating dairy (lactose), wheat and rye (because of the fructans they contain, *not* gluten, which is a protein), legumes (all beans, peas, chickpeas and lentils), most sweeteners, and many fruits and vegetables (including onions and garlic, apples, pears, melons, stone fruits, broccoli, cauliflower, and many others that are high in healthful soluble fiber like avocado, mushrooms, and beets). In fact, the justification for these global restrictions is that restricting just one type of FODMAP food (e.g. dairy or fructose alone) doesn't work because you really have to restrict *all* of them simultaneously. The FODMAP diet does allow *some* fruits (like bananas, citrus and blueberries) and vegetables (including carrots, eggplant, corn, celery and lettuce). But overall, it tends to be fairly meat heavy and fairly low fiber, which is ironic given all the evidence about the importance of eating a low meat, high fiber diet. It's really hard to stick to if you're a vegetarian, because it eliminates all the legumes and dairy (you can still eat eggs).

There is mounting evidence that following a low FODMAP diet can reduce discomfort and improve quality of life in IBD patients, especially if they have secondary IBS and the IBD is in remission.[29] One short-term study that lasted six weeks suggested that strict adherence to the low FODMAP diet could improve both patient reported symptoms and objective inflammatory markers in the stool.[30] BUT! There are some important caveats. First, the effect of restricting high FODMAP foods on the microbiome is worrisome. Whole species of "good" bacteria die out because they starve to death. Second, it's such a restrictive diet it's really quite hard to follow, and it's hard to get adequate nutrition on it under the best of circumstances. Even Peter Gibson, one of the originators of the diet, warns that "The risk of compromising nutritional status with a restrictive diet must be seriously considered especially as undernutrition is already common in this patient population ... As undernutrition is common in IBD, the use of restrictive diets should be supervised by a dietitian."[31] It's also important to note that you should never stick to the strict elimination phase of the diet for more than six weeks, for all the reasons listed above. You're supposed to start slowly reintroducing FODMAP containing foods over time until you get back to a reasonably varied diet.

The main problem with this diet from the perspective of the CBT approach is that it is really the mother of all avoidance strategies. Following this diet aims to reduce or eliminate many of the sensations that folks with chronic GI problems have become hypersensitive to. The goal of the program in this book is to reduce the hypersensitivity so you can eat whatever you want.

Fasting

In some ways, the most extreme restriction is intentional fasting. That is, don't eat at all for a set period of time. Lots of IBD patients try this at least some of the time. If you have a presentation at work, or you have to drive your daughter to a swim meet several hours away, it can be tempting to simply skip breakfast and lunch all together to limit the possibility of having to go to the bathroom. This is understandable, but it's really not a very good solution. Imagine if I told you that I had a treatment for IBD symptoms that worked really well short term. Alas, however, it has some unfortunate side effects. It will make you weak and dizzy and more easily fatigued. You might well get a headache or feel light-headed. It will slow your reaction time and impair your decision making, memory and impulse control. It will also probably make you irritable and more emotionally reactive. Sounds pretty terrible, right? Well, that's hunger for you. Low blood sugar will do all of those things. Remember that fasting is really an avoidance strategy. If you're still fasting regularly to try to reduce or avoid GI symptoms and bathroom trips, go back to Chapter 7 on eliminating avoidance and see if you can come up with some graded exposures to reintroduce more regular meals back into your routine.

Summary

In summary, there may be some foods that don't agree with you, at least some of the time, and there may be some strategies that will help you keep your gut functioning smoothly, efficiently and regularly. But there are also a lot of myths out there, and following ALL the advice out there on diet and GI problems will lead to an unnecessarily limited diet which compromises nutrition and lots of unnecessary anxiety about "DANGEROUS" trigger foods. During an active flare, you should almost certainly severely limit insoluble fiber and high residue foods, as your doctor will probably advise. When *not* in active flare, you may want to limit insoluble fiber somewhat and emphasize soluble fiber instead. But beyond that basic recommendation, there is very little evidence that dietary changes (especially highly restrictive diets) will help improve your IBD symptoms long term. Indeed, eating a diet that is too restrictive is likely to contribute to malnutrition and weight loss. To recap:

- Eating a typical Western diet that is meat heavy, high in saturated fat, high fructose corn syrup and/or fake sugar and processed foods, and low in fiber, fruits and vegetables isn't a good idea for anyone, and can increase the risk of developing an IBD and worsen the disease course if you already have an IBD. Aim to eat a highly varied diet rich in natural (not processed) foods, including whole grains, fruits and vegetables, and organic, humanely pasture raised sources of animal products (like dairy, eggs, and meat, if you eat it).
- Limiting insoluble fiber (from bran and fibrous vegetables) is probably a good idea and may be especially important during active flares.
- Consuming more *soluble* fiber is probably a good idea and should help reduce diarrhea. Eating a balanced diet in which you combine soluble and moderate amounts of insoluble fiber at every meal is probably the best strategy.
- Eliminating or strictly limiting high residue foods may be medically indicated and important during active flares, especially if you have strictures and are vulnerable to small bowel obstruction. This would include drastically reducing the amount of insoluble fiber you eat and would also mean temporarily eliminating foods like nuts, popcorn and celery that stay in chunks or form stringy tangles. However, the low-residue diet is not a general long-term strategy and you may incorporate these foods back into your diet as soon as your doctor tells you it is safe to do so.
- Limiting dairy products is unlikely to help, unless you're lactose intolerant. Even then, consuming fermented dairy (like yogurt or kefir), or aged cheese or using Lactaid products will allow you to get the calcium, protein and vitamin D you need for strong bones and muscles.
- Limiting wheat and other sources of gluten is unlikely to help unless you really have co-morbid Celiac Disease.
- Adding probiotics to your diet, either in the form of yogurt or in nutritional supplements, may indeed help, if your doctor okays it.

- Peppermint oil supplements may help relax the smooth muscles in your colon.
- Ginger can reduce nausea, but is unlikely to help most people with an IBD.
- Foods that tend to produce gas (like beans, soy foods and broccoli) are perfectly safe to eat, but many people (including people without GI problems) find that Beano reduces uncomfortable gas and flatulence.
- Eliminating fruit from your diet is impractical and unwise. By all means, however, cut out sodas and other processed foods that contain lots of high fructose corn syrup, and limit your exposure to "fake" sugars like sorbitol and xylitol.
- The FODMAP diet, which tries to eliminate a wide range of foods containing carbohydrates that may be poorly absorbed (including lactose and fructose), is a complex diet that requires the guidance of a registered dietician to follow safely. It involves eliminating a very wide range of foods including dairy, most grains, all the legumes, many fruits and vegetables and sweeteners and is *very* restrictive and difficult to follow. It may work to reduce symptoms in individuals with secondary IBS, but such an overly restrictive diet can compromise nutrition and should not be attempted by most people with an IBD. It can contribute to malnutrition and weight loss, and should *never* be attempted without the guidance of a registered dietician.
- Coffee stimulates colonic motility in just about everyone. If you find, after testing it systematically, that it worsens your cramping and diarrhea, don't drink it. You'll probably be better off.
- There is no evidence that meat or egg yolks contribute to intestinal distress in people with IBDs or IBS. Treating them as "dangerous" just contributes to the perception that the world of food is an unsafe place. Eat meat in moderation. If you can, buy grass fed, organic beef and organic cage free chickens. Buy organic eggs, but don't throw out the yolks! You deprive yourself of most of the wonderful nutrition nature put into those perfect little packages.
- Very greasy, fried food isn't good for anyone. Eat it infrequently and only in very small quantities.
- Many savory, tasty dishes are just fine to eat. There is a little bit of data suggesting that chili peppers may aggravate intestinal cramping and pain in people with secondary IBS, but there's also (a little) evidence that capsaicin may have anti-inflammatory properties that are helpful for folks with IBDs.
- Always follow your doctor's advice about specific dietary restrictions when your disease is active. If you're unsure why your doctor is making a particular recommendation, ask!

In the end, your goal should be to establish a balanced, tasty and *nutritious* diet for yourself that is relatively high in fruits and vegetables (peeled and cooked if you're in flare), legumes (taken with Beano), nut butters and some whole grains (with a bit more emphasis on oats and rice than wheat and corn), contains lots of heart healthy fats (from nuts, canola and olive oils), includes a reasonable portion of animal protein which can include fish, dairy, whole eggs, and meat of all kinds (unless you prefer a vegetarian diet for other reasons), *in moderation*, and is generally low in processed foods, caffeine and nutritionally "empty" calories from soda and candy. Avoid "fake" foods like olestra and artificial sweeteners. Do all this, and you optimize your chances of getting adequate nutrition without contributing to GI distress. Your heart, your waistline and your gut will all thank you.

Notes

1 Green, N., Miller, T., Suskind, D. & Lee, D. (2019). A review of dietary therapy for IBD and a vision for the future. *Nutrients*, 11(5), 947. https://doi.org/10.3390/nu11050947.

2 Knight-Sepulveda, K., Kais, S., Santaolalla, R. & Abreu, M.T. (2015). Diet and inflammatory bowel disease. *Gastroenterology & Hepatology*, 11(8), 511–520.

3 Hou, J.K., Lee, D. & Lewis, J. (2014). Diet and inflammatory bowel disease: Review of patient-targeted recommendations. *Clinical Gastroenterology and Hepatology*, 12, 1592–1600.

4 Yelencich, E., Truong, E., Widaman, A.M. et al. (2020). Risk of Avoidant/Restrictive Food Intake disorder (ARFID) is associated with impaired nutritional status in patients with inflammatory bowel diseases. *AGA Abstracts*, 158(6) S1. S–159.

5 Fernandez-Banares, F., Hinojosa, J., Sanchez-Lombrana, L. et al. (1999). Randomized clinical trial of Plantago ovata seeds (dietary fiber) as compared with mesalamine in maintaining remission in ulcerative colitis. *American Journal of Gastroenterology*, 94, 427–433.

6 Galvez, J., Rodriguez-Cabezas, M. & Zarzuelo, A. (2005). Effects of dietary fiber on inflammatory bowel disease. *Molecular Nutrition and Food Research*, 49, 601–608.

7 Olendzki, Silverstein, Persuitte, Ma, et al. (2014). An anti-inflammatory diet as treatment for inflammatory bowel disease: a case series report. *BMC: Nutrition Journal*, 13, Article 5.

8 Pituch-Zdanowska, Banaszkiewicz & Albrecht (2015). The role of dietary fiber in inflammatory bowel disease. *Prz Gastroenterol, 10(3)*, 135–141.

9 Von Tirpitz, C., Kohn, C., Steinkamp, M. et al. (2002). Lactose intolerance in active Crohn's disease: Clinical value of duodenal lactase analysis. *Journal of Clinical Gastroenterology*, 34(1), 49–53; Eadala, P., Matthews, S.B., Waud, J.P., Green, J.T. & Campbell, A.K. (2011) Association of lactose sensitivity with inflammatory bowel disease – demonstrated by analysis of genetic polymorphism, breath gases and symptoms. *Alimentary Pharmacology and Therapeutics*, 34, 735–746.

10 Szilagyi, A., Galiatsatos, P. & Xue, X. (2015). Systematic review and meta-analysis of lactose digestion, its impact on intolerance and nutritional effects of dairy food restriction in inflammatory bowel disease. *Nutrition Journal*, 13, Article 67.

11 Shah, A., Walker, M., Burder, D. et al. (2019). Link between celiac disease and inflammatory bowel disease. *Journal of Clinical Gastroenterology*, 53(7), 514–522.

12 Derwa, Y., Gracie, D.J., Hamlin, P.J. & Ford, A.C. (2017). Systematic review with meta-analysis: the efficacy of probiotics in inflammatory bowel disease. *Alimentary Pharmacology and Therapeutics*, 46, 389–400. https://doi.org/10.1111/apt.14203; Abraham, B.P. & Quigley, E.M.M. (2017). Probiotics in inflammatory bowel disease. *Gastroenterology Clinics of North America*, 46, 769–782.

13 Ciorba, M.A. (2012). A gastroenterologist's guide to probiotics. *Clinical Gastroenterology and Hepatology*, 10(9), 960–968. https://dx.doi.org/10.1016%2Fj.cgh.2012.03.024.

14 Chumpitazi, B.P., Kearns, G. & Shulman, R.J. (2018). Review article: The physiologic effects and safety of Peppermint Oil and its efficacy in irritable bowel

syndrome and other functional disorders. *Alimentary Pharmacology and Therapeutics*, 47 (6), 738–752. https://dx.doi.org/10.1111%2Fapt.14519.

15 Cappello, G., Spezzaferro, M., Grossi, L., Manzoli, L. & Marzio, L. (2007). Peppermint oil (Mintoil) in the treatment of irritable bowel syndrome: A prospective double blind placebo-controlled randomized trial. *Digestive and Liver Disease*, 39, 530–536.

16 Shams, R., Oldfield, E.C., Copare, J. & Johnson, D.A. (2015). Peppermint oil: Clinical uses in the treatment of gastrointestinal diseases. *JSM Gastroenterology and Hepatology*, 3(1), 1035.

17 El-Aghar, H.S., Hammad, L. & Gawad, H.S.A. (2008). Modulating effect of ginger extract on rats with ulcerative colitis. *Journal of Ethnopharmacology*, 118(3), 367–372.

18 Shayesteh, F., Haidari, R., Shayesteh, A.A., Mohammadi-Asl, J. & Ahmadi-Angali, K. (2020). Ginger in patients with active ulcerative colitis: a study protocol for a randomized controlled trial. *BMC Trials*, 21, 278. https://doi.org/10.1186/s13063-020-4193-7.

19 DiStefano, M., Miceli, E., Gotti, S., Missanelli, A., Mazzocchi, S. & Corazza, G.R. (2007). The effect of oral alpha-galactosidase on intestinal gas production and gas-related symptoms. *Digestive Diseases and Sciences*, 52(1), 78–83.

20 Barrett, J.S., Irving, P.M., Shepherd, S.J. et al. (2009). Comparison of the prevalence of fructose and lactose malabsorption across chronic intestinal disorders. *Alimentary Pharmacology & Therapeutics*, 30(2), 165–174.

21 Ruiz-Ojeda, F.J., Plaza-Diaz, J., Saez-Lara, M.J. & Gil, A. (2019). Effects of sweeteners on the gut microbiota: A review of experimental studies and clinical trials. *Advances in Nutrition*, 10(S1), S31–S48. https://dx.doi.org/10.1093%2Fadvances%2Fnmy037.

22 Rao, S.S., Welcher, K., Zimmerman, B. & Stumbo, P. (1998). Is coffee a colonic stimulant? *European Journal of Gastroenterology*, 10, 113–118.

23 Barthel, C. Wiegand, S. Scharl, S. et al. (2015). Patients' perceptions on the impact of coffee consumption in inflammatory bowel disease: friend or foe? – a patient survey. *Nutritional Journal*, 14, 78.

24 Jaquet, M., Rochat, I., Moulin, J. et al. (2009). Impact of coffee consumption on the gut microbiota: A human volunteer study. *International Journal of Food Microbiology*, 130(2), 117–121.

25 Hou, J., Abraham, B. & Hashem, E.L. (2011). Dietary intake and risk of developing inflammatory bowel disease: A systematic review of the literature. *American Journal of Gastroenterology*, 106(4), 563–573.

26 Tasson, L., Canova, C., Vettorato, M.G., Savarino, E. & Zanotti, R. (2017). Influence of diet on the course of inflammatory bowel disease. *Digestive Diseases and Sciences*, 62, 2087–2094.

27 Akbar, A., Yiangou, Y., Facer, P., Walters, J.R.F, Anand, P. & Ghosh, S. (2008). Increased capsaicin receptor TRPV1-expressing sensory fibres in irritable bowel syndrome and their correlation with abdominal pain. *Gut*, 57, 923–929.

28 Dos Santos, E.A. & Alvarez-Leite, J.I. (2019). Capsaicin: A potential therapy adjuvant for intestinal bowel disease. *Journal of Digestive disorders and Diagnosis*, https://doi.org/10.14302/issn.2574-4526.jddd-19-3063.

29 Prince, A.C., Myers, C.E., Joyce, T. Irving, P. Lomer, M. & Whelan, K. (2016). Fermentable carbohydrate restrictions (low FODMAP diet) in clinical practice improves functional gastrointestinal symptoms in patients with inflammatory bowel disease. *Inflammatory Bowel Diseases*, 22(5), 1129–1136; Pederson, N., Ankersen, D. V., Felding, M., Wachmann, H., Vegh, Z., Molzen, L., Burisch, J., Anderson, J.R. & Munkholm, P. (2017). Low-FODMAP diet reduces irritable bowel symptoms in patients with inflammatory bowel disease. *World Journal of Gastroenterology*, 23(18), 356–3366; Testa, A., Imperatore, N., Rispo, A., Rea, M., Tortora, R., Nardone, O.M., Lucci, L., Accarino, G., Caporaso, N. & Castiglione, F. (2018). Beyond

irritable bowel syndrome: The efficacy of the low FODMAP diet for improving symptoms in inflammatory bowel diseases and celiac disease. *Digestive Diseases*, 36(4), 271–280.

30 Bodini, G., Zanella, C., Crespi, M., Lo Pumo, S., Demarzo, M.G., Savarino, E., Savarino, V. & Giannini, E.G. (2019). A randomized, 6-week trial of a low FODMAP diet in patients with inflammatory bowel disease. *Nutrition*, 67–68, https://doi.org/10.1016/j.nut.2019.06.023.

31 Gibson, P.R. (2017). Use of the low-FODMAP diet in inflammatory bowel disease. *Journal of Gastroenterology and Hepatology*.https://doi.org/10.1111/jgh.13695.

9 Thinking About Medical Management

Medical management of your IBD is the domain of expertise of your gastro-enterologist and other physicians and this chapter is not intended in any way to replace the advice of your doctor. The goal of this chapter is to help you think through some of the common fears patients with an IBD might have about medical management, and coping strategies that might help. We'll touch on five major areas: managing the doctor/patient relationship; scopes and other diagnostic techniques; steroids, which most IBD patients have a love/hate relationship with; other medication options; and surgery.

The Doctor/Patient Relationship

First, a few words about building a trusting, collaborative relationship with your gastroenterologist. It's incredibly important. You need to establish with your doctor how you prefer to manage your care. Do you want detailed explanations of the treatment options with all their potential risks and benefits so that you can make an informed decision? Some people love that. If you're one of them, be sure you establish a respectful relationship with a doctor who wants to educate you and takes your opinions and preferences seriously. Or are you someone who wants your doctor (who is the expert who went to medical school, after all!) to make clear recommendations without burdening you with too much detailed information that might feel overwhelming and hard to understand? Be sure to tell your doctor that. Maybe you just want to ask about potential side effects so you can be reassured and have your fears set to rest. Maybe you don't even want to hear about the laundry list of potential adverse effects because it's too scary, and what's the point? Any and all of these coping styles are legitimate and appropriate, if they are what work for you. But you may need to educate your doctor about what you need from them.

Doctors are incredibly busy and have many demands on their time and attention. But that's no excuse for not taking the time to answer your questions and respond to your concerns. It's a good idea to have a list of questions and concerns on paper (or in your phone) when you go to your appointment. This will help you remember what you want to ask in a short amount of time and will provide some structure to the appointment. It can be hard to remember

DOI: 10.4324/9781003057635-10

what you wanted to talk about when you're being hit with recent test results or new treatment options. But things will inevitably come up in the appointment that you don't have time or the focus to ask about further. Lots of hospital systems have online systems that let you communicate securely with your doctor via email. Take advantage of it!

If you feel that your doctor is being dismissive or rude, or isn't taking your concerns seriously, the first thing to do is to talk to them about it. Explain, briefly and respectfully, that you know they are busy, but you need a bit more time to ask questions and make sure you understand everything. The vast majority of doctors are truly decent, caring human beings who want to provide compassionate care. They're just overwhelmed at times. But if you try to talk to your doctor and you still feel uncomfortable or unhappy with your care, it may be time to try to find a new doctor. This can be hard outside of big cities with several major medical centers, but finding a doctor you feel comfortable with, who respects you, takes their time, and answers your questions, is a really important part of managing your IBD.

Of course, this works both ways! Part of collaborating effectively with your doctor means that you also have to communicate in a clear and timely way *with them*. If you have recently started a new medication, or have undergone a diagnostic procedure, you should call your doctor as soon as *anything* seems to be going wrong. Even if the side effects aren't serious, you should let your doctor make sure they aren't indicative of something more concerning. Even if you have been on a medicine for a while, you should always let your doctor know if there is a change in your symptoms or your experience. *You* are an incredibly important member of your treatment team. Many people hesitate to pick up the phone and let their doctor know when something doesn't feel right. People often think to themselves, "I don't want to bother him or her or waste his or her time. I don't want to be *that* patient who complains or is seen as whiny or bothersome or wimpy." Let me tell you right now that this drives doctors *crazy*! No physician in their right mind would be bothered by a patient calling in about a genuine alteration in symptoms or sensations. They *want* you to keep them informed in a timely way about the course of your treatment. If you don't call them, they are left in the dark and can't provide excellent care, and that frustrates them more than anything. A problem that would be minor if caught right away can become major if it's left unmanaged. Trust me, your doctor would *much* rather hear from you right away than find out days later that a problem has escalated and is now going to be much more complicated to fix. So be an MVP on your own treatment team and keep your doctor in the loop with what's happening!

Communicating with your doctor also means being honest and transparent with them about a number of things, including embarrassing symptoms (like fecal incontinence or sexual issues) and issues related to taking medication as prescribed. Lots of patients forget to take their medicine at the right time. Or hesitate to take the full dose. Or fill the scrip but don't take the medication at all. If you've ever done any of these things, it's really important to be honest with your doctor about it. They can't make reasonable decisions about whether a treatment is working if they don't know what you're actually doing. You should frame the conversation in a way that makes clear what your concerns are about following the protocol you've been prescribed. If you have lingering doubts or worries about the safety or efficacy of a medication, or you don't understand what the medication is supposed to do or why the medication is being prescribed in the way that it is, ask! You may feel guilty or be worried that the doctor is going to "yell" at you for not following directions. A good doctor might express some frustration or disappointment, but they should pivot pretty quickly to addressing your concerns. Remember this is your body, and your doctor is your partner in managing your care. You need to work *together* to make that care happen.

Scopes, MREs and Cameras

Many IBD patients will need to undergo diagnostic or imaging procedures periodically to facilitate diagnosis, and to monitor their IBD and figure out whether the management strategies are working. There are three basic kinds of diagnostic procedures beyond the blood work and stool tests that can check for inflammatory markers in, you guessed it, blood and stool. Scopes (endoscopy and colonoscopy) both involve inserting a tube with a light, a camera, and a tool for taking biopsies into the digestive tract, either through the mouth (endoscopy) or the anus (colonoscopy). Imaging studies (such as magnetic resonance enterography or MRE and computed tomography or CT scans) are non-invasive and take pictures from outside the body. They can be used to image parts of the bowel that the scopes can't get to. Imaging can be used to distinguish UC from CD at the time of initial diagnosis; to assess and track progression of extraintestinal IBD manifestations; to visualize penetrating complications of disease that extend outside the bowel wall (like fistulas); and to assess disease activity in patients with known IBD during symptomatic recurrence (including checking for strictures and abscesses).[1] Finally, in capsule endoscopy, you swallow a vitamin pill sized camera, which takes pictures of your entire digestive tract as it goes through the system, transmitting the digital images to a small receiver you wear on a belt at your waist.

The hardest part of a colonoscopy is undoubtedly the prep. Your gut needs to be *empty* in order for the doctor to get a clear view of your intestines and take tissue samples (biopsies) for examination in the lab. That means you have to stop eating high residue foods a few days before the procedure. The day before the procedure you typically won't be allowed to eat any solid food at all. Clear liquids including broth, water, ice, sports drinks (but no red or purple food color) are typically allowed. Then the worst part is taking the bowel "prep," which is typically a laxative (a *lot* of laxative) such as Miralax. For some folks with IBD, having watery diarrhea is so common that it feels like no big deal. For others, the prep – and having hours of urgent watery diarrhea – is exhausting and awful. Even if it feels like no big deal to you, be sure not to schedule anything the day of the prep or the procedure. It's a good idea to take two full days off. You will also need a responsible adult to give you a ride to and from the procedure.

Some doctors' offices will instruct you to start the prep around 6 pm the night before the procedure. They typically recommend this so that you could, in theory, work the day before the procedure. The problem with this for many people is that then they will be up until 2 or 3 in the morning on and off the toilet. This can really interfere with sleep (obviously) and make the whole thing more exhausting than it needs to be. If you don't plan to work the day before the procedure, ask your doctor about starting the prep around noon instead. That way you'll be completely done pooping by bedtime, and can get a good night's rest. It's a good idea to schedule the procedure for first thing in the morning, if your doctor is available. That way you can eat afterwards and not spend the whole morning feeling weak and hungry, waiting to go have it done.

If you've never had a scope done, be assured that it is almost always done under a short acting form of general anesthesia, so that you have no awareness of the procedure itself. It usually wears off immediately, so you should feel awake and alert relatively quickly when it's done. If you have a history of difficulty shaking off anesthesia, you may feel dizzy and loopy for a few hours. That's part of why it's important to have someone pick you up and drive you home. And really, be kind to yourself. Don't try to work or do any chores for the rest of the day. Eat, drink (not alcohol!), and take the day to recover and recoup your energy.

Sometimes patients have catastrophic fears about what might happen during a scope. While complications are not unheard of, they are very, very rare. While it is theoretically possible that the scope will perforate the wall of the bowel, or that a biopsy site will bleed profusely, or that you'll somehow pick up a C. diff infection during the procedure, your doctor should assure you that in the vast majority of cases things go very smoothly and no adverse events occur. For example, perforations occur in far less than 0.1% of colonoscopies, and the majority of those occur in elderly patients, or patients who have very large polyps removed. (The largest study to date looked at close to three million procedures, and found a perforation rate of 0.016%.) While perforations can be dangerous, if they are caught right away they can typically be treated quickly and without long-term negative effects. If you have an experienced gastroenterologist doing the procedure, you should relax and know that you are in good hands.[2]

The prep for an endoscopy, MRE or CT scan is much easier. For an endoscopy, you stop eating and drinking by midnight the night before the procedure. For an MRE or CT, typically, you don't eat anything for about four to six hours before the procedure. For both types of scan, you will typically drink a "contrast" solution before entering the scanner. The hardest part of the MRE for most people is the time you spend inside the scanner. You lie on a gurney which then slides into a large tube. People who are prone to claustrophobia often find this quite unnerving. In addition, the machine is quite loud when it's taking the pictures. You have to lie there without moving in a relatively narrow tube with loud noises pounding away. I strongly suggest closing your eyes, and using your deep breathing and imagery skills. Imagine you're at the beach. Breathe slowly. Do a meditative body scan.

Remember that claustrophobia is the result of you imagining terrible things that aren't actually happening. Then your body responds to the scary images by triggering your fight or flight response. Now you're imagining scary things and all the feedback from your body is telling you that you're really scared, which seems to confirm that something terrible is happening, and you'd better get out of there. But it all started because you were imagining something that wasn't really happening. Bears and bats don't get claustrophobia because they don't *imagine* scary counterfactual things happening, like the cave they're in collapsing on them, or the entrance getting blocked off and not being able to breathe. Only humans get claustrophobia, because only humans *imagine* all kinds of terrible things, like being trapped or buried alive. Imagination, and the ability to visualize things that don't exist, is our human superpower. It's what produces great literature and indoor plumbing and landed humans on the moon. It's a great thing when we use it effectively. But it gets us into trouble when we use it for the powers of evil – imagining terrifying things that frighten us and get our heart pounding and our palms sweating. Instead, use your imagination for the power of good. Let it take you away from this annoying noisy tube. Either focus on your breathing, or imagine a safe, relaxing place, like the beach or the woods. Just like you learned in Chapter 3, make it as real as you can, engaging all the senses. Or try to remember all the lyrics to your favorite songs. Even reviewing the multiplication tables in your head can be distracting. If you give your mind something better to focus on, it won't have time to take you someplace scary, and your MRE will be a walk in the park (at least in your imagination!).

The worst thing that can happen with a capsule endoscopy is that the camera will get "stuck" inside you (technically called capsule retention) rather than coming out in a poop. This is only likely if you have significant strictures or scarring at the site of an anastomosis, or serious ulcerations. If that happens, the capsule will have to be removed, either with endoscopy or surgery, depending on where it got stuck. Often a doctor will have an IBD patient do a CT scan first to check for possible strictures where the capsule might get lodged. Fortunately, the capsules are getting smaller all the time as the technology improves. There are also procedures your doctor can use to check to see if a capsule will make it through even if you have strictures (called an agile patency system, it uses a dissolvable capsule first and you only use the real capsule if that one makes it through). Moreover, capsule retention is less likely if the GI center is experienced with the procedure. As always, having a GI doc you really trust and can talk through all these risks with is golden and can make you feel much more comfortable about undergoing these procedures.

Steroids

Love 'em or hate 'em, steroids are going to be part of medical management at some point for most patients with an IBD. The two main steroids that would be likely to be prescribed to someone with an IBD are prednisone and budesonide (Entocort or Uceris). Both have significant anti-inflammatory effects while you are taking them. They can calm down symptomatic flares and improve your GI symptoms significantly, typically inducing remission in a relatively short period of time. This is the "love 'em" part of steroids. Unfortunately, steroids only work while you're taking them, and they have a lot of side effects, so they should generally only be used in the lowest effective dose for the shortest amount of time possible. Prednisone can be helpful for both Crohn's and UC whereas budesonide is typically used in Crohn's because it is effective at the end of the small intestine (ilieum) and the beginning of the colon (cecum). There is a new form of budesonide (Uceris) that can also be used in UC.

It's important to remember that nearly every drug in existence, including aspirin, carries an enormous laundry list of potential side effects, ranging from mildly annoying to downright terrifying. Unfortunately, there is usually no way for your doctor to predict exactly which side effects, if any, will occur, and how severe they will be. Different people may react in completely different ways to the same drug. The only way to know how *you* will react is if *you* take the drug. The important thing is to evaluate the risk/benefit profile of any given treatment option objectively, without catastrophizing all the possibilities.

About half of people taking steroids will experience a particular side effect called "moon face" in which the face swells up (due to fatty deposits in the cheeks and temples) and looks much rounder than normal. Doctors consider this a "minor" side effect because it's not dangerous and it usually resolves within a few weeks to a month when you stop taking the drug. But most patients *hate* it. It's embarrassing. You don't look like yourself. People might ask you about it. Lots of people say it makes them feel "fat" even when their overall weight hasn't changed. So while doctors might not worry about it because it's just "cosmetic" (not dangerous) patients are often quite distressed by it. My advice is two-fold. First, remember that it is temporary. Second, if people ask you about it, just tell them the truth!

More "serious" side effects of steroids can include nervousness or agitation, slightly worsening depression, mood swings, greater vulnerability to infections, and long-term osteoporosis or weakened bones. This is the real "hate 'em" side of steroids, and it's why you want to be on them at the lowest dose for the shortest time that you can manage. That said, steroids can dramatically improve your quality of life, and can give your gut a chance to calm down and heal, which can give other medications a chance to take effect. As with any choice, you have to weight the potential risks and benefits of both taking the steroid, *and* the potential risks and benefits of *not* taking the steroid. One of the advantages of budesonide (over prednisone) is that it tends to have fewer systemic (whole body) effects, and concentrates the effects in the intestines where it's needed, so your doctor will typically opt for that if he or she thinks it will be effective, reserving prednisone for more severe flares.

I like to remind my patients that if their doctor recommends short term use of steroids, they should go for it. Some people get so worried about long-term consequences (like osteoporosis) that they would rather endure severe pain, weight loss, fatigue and other symptoms rather than take the steroid. I remind people that this is faulty logic. If you're gut is badly inflamed, you're at high risk for nutritional deficiencies, which in itself puts you at higher risk for osteoporosis! I would much rather that people took the steroids for a time to get their IBD under better control in the short term. It can dramatically improve quality of life while you work with your doctor to come up with a good long-term solution that will help keep you in remission when you wean off the steroid.

Other Medications

The list of other medications that can be used to treat IBDs is long and ever changing, and even a comprehensive review would probably be out of date pretty quickly. So rather than going through each class and discussing their potential uses, mechanisms of action and side effects, I want to touch on the general emotional issues that might come up for people.

Mode of Delivery

Some IBD drugs must be taken as an injection or an infusion. This can mean going to a center to get the infusions, or learning to give oneself injections at home. For folks who don't have a background in medicine, this can be intimidating, but most people get the hang of it pretty quickly and it starts to seem routine. Other issues include pain or discomfort during the injection. Newer formulations of some drugs (like citrate free Humira) have dramatically reduced the burning pain many people associated with the injection. This has been a huge boon to IBD patients everywhere.

Actual Delivery

Other drugs need to be delivered by post from mail-order pharmacies. Some need to be kept cold (like Stelara) and if you work outside the home it may be tricky to figure out when to have it delivered so that someone can get it into the fridge as soon as possible. Rest assured that this (expensive) drug won't be spoiled even if the cold chain is briefly interrupted. It keeps for 30 days. So try not to fret too much if it ends up sitting on your front porch for a few hours until you get home.

Potential Side Effects

Many of the powerful drugs used to treat IBD have potential side effects that can be scary or even life threatening. Many patients are reluctant to even try a medication because of the possibility (however slight) of liver or kidney toxicity, infection, or even cancer. Those concerns are real, and you need to discuss with your doctor what steps can be taken to minimize the chances of experiencing these adverse effects. For example, doctors will typically want to monitor kidney and/or liver health with regular blood work, and may decide to adjust the dose, or switch to a new medicine entirely if there are issues. As always, you need to consider not just the risks of taking the drug, but also the risks of *not* taking the drug. Several IBD drugs increase the risk of skin cancer in particular. You can minimize this risk by wearing sunscreen and visiting your dermatologist yearly to get checked. Remember that untreated IBD itself can increase your risk of colon cancer significantly. So you have to take your total cancer risk into account in making your decisions. If your quality of life is really taking a beating because your IBD isn't under good control, then not pursuing your medical options out of fear of *potential* side effects is probably unwise.

One thing we know about how people tend to think about risk is that most people are much more upset about the thought of *doing* something that ends up having a bad result than they are about *not doing* something that ends up having a bad result. Technically called errors of commission, we don't like *committing acts* that we end up regretting. Weirdly, errors of omission (failing to act) don't usually stir up quite the same feelings of guilt and regret. It's odd, because failing to act can have consequences that are just as bad. So people tend to worry a lot more about deciding to *take* Remicade or Stelara, and then regretting it because they developed an adverse effect, than they worry about deciding *not* to manage their IBD aggressively, and having bad outcomes as a result. Even though this bias towards judging sins of commission more harshly is pretty universal, it's actually pretty illogical. They are both choices to behave in a certain way that end up having consequences.

Lots of folks with an IBD are tough – they can tolerate a lot of discomfort, fatigue, skin lesions, joint pain, diarrhea, you name it. I have tremendous respect for people who manage to go about their lives (even if in a somewhat limited way) carrying the burdens of an active IBD. But I strongly encourage my patients to consider their overall quality of life when making decisions about medication management. If medication can drastically improve your quality of life, it's almost certainly worth giving it a try.

It's also worth remembering that new medications are being developed and tested for inflammatory bowel diseases every day. Sometimes new medicines become available in limited ways to people in clinical trials or through special restricted distribution programs. Sometimes, it isn't clear whether the benefits of a medication will outweigh the risks associated with using it. Obviously, you will want a doctor who stays abreast of all the latest developments in medicines for IBDs and who will help you think through clearly the potential costs and benefits *for you* of any particular medication regimen, given the type and severity of your IBD, the location of the inflammation, the impact of the IBD on your quality of life and overall health and so on. We can all fervently hope that new drug discoveries are on the horizon that will bring a true cure. This isn't just wishful thinking. After all, ten years ago Hepatitis C was considered hard to treat and almost impossible to cure – and the medication regimens that existed had terrible side effects for lots of people who tried them (including suicidal depression – yikes!). Today there are several medications that can cure up to 98% of patients with Hepatitis C and have *very* benign side effect profiles. It's really amazing when you think about it. So keep asking your doctor about new trials and new developments. Maybe one day soon we'll be able to cure IBDs too, without the risk of serious side effects.

Surgeries

About 20% of patient with ulcerative colitis and up to 50% of Crohn's patients will eventually need surgery of some sort. Considering the high likelihood, you should have a long conversation with your doctor about possible surgical options, even if only to plan ahead. The most important caveat about surgery is that it doesn't "cure" Crohn's – Crohn's is an autoimmune disease, and is not localized in any part of the gut. However, surgery can provide dramatic symptom relief, and with proper medication management further surgery may never be necessary. Most doctors wish that their IBD patients would be willing to consider surgery sooner rather than later. A lot of people delay surgery, sometimes for years, while they continue to suffer. They're in pain, having complications, missing school or work. Surgery can make a dramatic difference to quality of life and many people then wonder why they waited so long.

While surgery will almost never be the first option, there are many situations in which surgery will become absolutely necessary. These include:

- *Severe strictures*, which are sections of the digestive tract that have become scarred by repeated inflammation. The walls of these sections will thicken and form scar tissue, which will narrow that section of the intestine, increasing the risk of intestinal blockage. Surgery can be used to remove or widen a segment of intestine that has become too narrow.
- *Small bowel obstruction*, which occurs when food becomes stuck or lodged in the intestines (usually at a point of a stricture). This is a medical emergency, and surgery to clear the obstruction (and typically to widen the stricture) can be life-saving in this situation if the obstruction fails to respond to medical therapy.
- *Intestinal bleeding*, which is thankfully rare in IBD. Mild cases can be managed by medication, but severe cases will require surgery.
- *Perforations*, which are holes in the wall of the digestive tract that form after the tissue has been weakened by inflammation.

- *Fistulas*, which occur when an ulcer (sore) forms in the wall of the digestive tract and extends to another part of the body, either another part of the digestive tract or another organ. This creates a hole between these two organs, allowing material to leak through. Drugs such as TNF inhibitors can be used to close fistulas. However, if these are ineffective then surgery is required to close them.
- *Abscesses*, which are painful pockets of pus that must be surgically drained.
- *Toxic megacolon*, which is a sudden swelling of the colon that causes toxins to leak into the blood.

Surgery may also be needed if medical therapy fails for patients with severe disease who can no longer bear the symptoms. The full list of risks and complications associated with various surgeries are far beyond the scope of this book, and vary significantly from patient to patient. If your doctor recommends surgery, you should have a long, in-depth conversation with your surgeon about the pros, cons, risks and potential benefits of any specific surgical treatment.

Summary

It is true that every medical approach to IBD has potential side effects or adverse consequences. This can be anxiety provoking and frustrating. It is also true that IBD *itself* has lots of negative effects, including potentially life-threatening ones. So managing your IBD proactively is smart and necessary. You can be the toughest, strongest, most resilient person on the planet, but if your body can't absorb nutrients from food, you're not going to be able to function anywhere near your best. Yes, some of the medications used to manage IBD increase your risk of infection and of certain cancers. But untreated IBD increases your risk of *other* cancers. So don't let fear of possible side effects or fear of the idea of surgery keep you from managing your IBD aggressively and proactively.

The bottom line is that medical management of your IBD is a complex, potentially life-long process that should ideally be a collaborative partnership between you and your trusted gastroenterologist. Talk to your doctor. Make sure your doctor understands how much you want to know and how the two of you will make decisions about your care. Make sure you communicate clearly to your doctor about your goals for treatment. With respectful, thoughtful, collaborative care, you get your best chance at living the full, rich life you want.

Notes

1 Kilcoyne, A., Kaplan, J.L. & Gee, M.S. (2016). Inflammatory bowel disease imaging: Current practice and future directions. *World Journal of Gastroentology*, 22(3), 917–932.
2 Kim, S.Y., Kim, H.S. & Park, H.J. (2019). Adverse events related to colonoscopy: Global trends and future challenges. *World Journal of Gastroenterology*, 25(2), 190–204.

10 What If I Need an Ostomy?

People who live with some type of ostomy procedure, or ostomates, are not uncommon among IBD patients. As medical management improves and new medications are developed, the rates of ostomy procedures are going down somewhat, but for some people with an IBD, either a temporary or permanent ostomy procedure may still be necessary. In this chapter, we will discuss the various types of equipment ostomates use as well as address the impact on daily activities and some common concerns.

What is an Ostomy and Why Would I Need One?

An ostomy is a surgically created opening in the body for the expulsion of waste. The opening itself is called a stoma. Stomas vary in size, shape, and location, but many patients say their stoma resembles a rosebud. It is usually placed in the lower quadrant of the abdomen somewhat off to the side.

Temporary Versus Permanent

Ostomies can be temporary or permanent. Surgeons might perform a temporary ostomy for a variety of reasons, such as when a patient has a perforation in the bowel and requires surgery. The temporary ostomy allows the surgery to heal without risk of contamination. Intestinal function can be restored to normal when the ostomy is reversed. Permanent ostomies are performed when a segment of the upper or lower intestine cannot be repaired. It is important to note that permanent ostomies are a surgery of last resort. They are performed on patients presenting with severe symptoms that can no longer be managed by medications.

Ileostomies Versus Colostomies

The two types of ostomies performed on patients with IBDs are ileostomies and colostomies. The main difference between the two is that an ileostomy involves the small intestine and a colostomy involves the large intestine. In an ileostomy, the end of the small intestine is brought through the abdominal wall

DOI: 10.4324/9781003057635-11

to form a stoma. There are many types of colostomies, and they vary based on the exact portion of the colon used to create the stoma.

Mourning and Adjustment

Learning to control one's bowels and urination are major developmental milestones for growing children, and are often a source of pride when accomplished, and distress when "accidents" happen as children get older. So let's take a moment to acknowledge that losing that control as an adult can be a real blow. You may need to take some time to "mourn" the loss of a normative body function. At times you might feel angry. At times you might feel very sad. There is no set pattern or timeline for how you "should" feel or when you should be feeling a particular way. The so-called "stages of grief" (denial, anger, bargaining, depression and acceptance) are a popular model, but there's actually very little empirical evidence that people experience any or all of these "stages" at all, much less in that particular order. Some people who decide to get an ostomy are so *relieved* that it will end their constant pain and debilitating symptoms that they are really just glad to put their active disease behind them. Nevertheless, most people will struggle with the decision somewhat, and may be experiencing a complex mix of feelings at any given point in time, including relief, anxiety, curiosity, dread, anger and plain old exhaustion. Going to a support group with experienced ostomates can often help allay some anxiety and can give you a place where it is completely "safe" to talk about your apprehension and get good advice about adjusting successfully to life with an ostomy.

The Ostomate's Toolkit

• Pouch system
• Pouch accessories

Pouching systems have three main functions: collect stool, contain odor, and protect the skin around the stoma from contact with waste.

Types of Pouching Systems

All pouching systems have a pouch to collect waste and something called a wafer, or skin barrier, that holds the pouch to the skin. In *one-piece systems*, the wafer is already attached to the pouch and in order to remove the pouch you must remove the wafer as well. In *two-piece systems*, the pouch and skin barrier are separate. The wafer in two-piece systems comes with a special rim called a flange that seals the pouch to the wafer. These systems also come in two varieties: open-end pouches and close-end pouches. *Open-end pouches* are drainable. In open-end systems, waste is expelled from the bottom of the bag. When the bag is not being emptied, the bottom is held secure by a clipping device. *Closed-end pouches* cannot be drained; when the pouch is full, it is discarded. Closed-end systems are used when the pouch doesn't have to be emptied often.

The *wafer/skin barrier* comes in many styles. There are flat models and convex models; rigid and flexible models; and models with and without adhesive backing.

Choosing a Pouching System

Because every stoma and every body is unique, different people will respond differently to different pouch systems and wafer types. New ostomates should try out different models and see what feels most comfortable. Being open to different systems is especially important for the period after surgery, when the size of the stoma will be changing as the swelling goes down.

There are some tips that can help narrow down the type of pouching systems and skin barriers you choose to try. Because ileostomies produce a more watery output than colostomies, the pouching systems need to be emptied more often. If you have an ileostomy, it may be more convenient for you to use an open-ended, drainable system and to use a larger sized pouch (to decrease the number of times the pouch must be drained during the day).

Although wear time for pouching systems varies, open-end pouches can generally be used for three to seven days, depending on the specific model (close-end pouches are, of course, designed for one time use). It might be helpful to keep in mind that both types of systems can have wear time decreased by factors such as perspiration and increased exposure to water (through activities like swimming).

Accessories

Specially constructed ostomy *belts* can be worn around the abdomen to provide increased support for the ostomy pouch. Some ostomates choose to wear belts in addition to adhesive skin barriers because they help keep a pouch in place and some ostomates use them in place of adhesive skin barriers. If you choose to wear a belt, be sure to abide by the "one finger rule" which states that you should be able to place one finger width between the belt and your abdomen. Following this rule helps protect you from making the belt too tight, causing cuts or grooves in the skin.

Pre-made *pouch covers* are also available (or you could do it yourself in fun patterns if you're handy with a sewing machine). Some ostomates prefer to use pouch covers daily to reduce the discomfort caused by the pouch coming into frequent contact with their skin. Many ostomates also choose to use pouch covers during intimate moments for coverage as well as to prevent friction if the pouch comes into contact with a partner's skin.

There are many commercial products available from medical supply companies and specialty websites like www.ostomysecrets.com that are actually quite attractive, pretty, cool and/or sexy. They sell belts, wraps, swim wraps and underwear (including briefs and boxers for men and sexy, lacy panties and even thongs for women) that will help you feel secure and attractive both clothed and during intimacy. Don't be afraid to shop around until you find the products that work for you.

Many ostomates, particularly new ostomates, can be uncomfortable with the scent of ostomy discharge, which is subtly and sometimes not so subtly different from the smell of regular feces. Although pouching systems have built-in deodorizers, there is no built-in odor control for when the pouch is being emptied. Additional *deodorizers* are available to control odor during pouch draining. These come in many forms including sprays for the pouch, tablets to be put into the pouch, and pills taken orally. The best way to see what works for you is to explore the various options. Of course, it's important to remember that *everybody's poop smells*. Even before you developed an IBD, your poop varied in the type of odor it produced. Everyone's does. Sometimes poop is especially stinky and sometimes it's not. *Anyone* who poops in a public restroom will leave some odor in their wake. This is normal, and nothing to be disgusted or shamed by. In fact, it's important to try not react with disgust or shame to your own body's waste. However unusual your stoma may be, waste is natural and normal.

One funny *advantage* to an ostomy is that some pouching systems have *filters* built in to allow gas to escape, and you can also purchase them separately and attach them to your pouching system. Filtering systems generally *deodorize* gas as it is expelled as well as prevent gas from causing a pressure buildup in the pouch. This means you get to filter your farts and no one needs to smell them ever again. People without ostomies don't have that option!

Maintenance

Emptying the Pouch

Many ostomates develop their own methods for emptying open-end pouches cleanly and efficiently. One common tip is to put toilet paper in the bowl before draining to avoid splash back. Some people prefer to empty the pouch in a standing position and some prefer to do so in a sitting position. Regardless of what makes you most comfortable, be sure to wipe the tip with toilet paper and put the clip back in place. As always, it is important to *normalize* your experience with this as much as possible. Before your ostomy you, like everyone else, used toilet paper or wet wipes to wipe the smeared poop off your bottom and from around your anus every time you defecated. This is simply part of normal life hygiene. You are now wiping an appliance rather than the skin around your anus and this is weird and different in some ways, but in many ways it is *not* that different. After some practice with it, it will come as naturally to you as wiping your bottom ever did, and you will be able to do it neatly and efficiently.

Changing Your Appliance

Pouching systems come with their own instructions for appliance changes, but here is a breakdown of the basic procedure. When the procedure differs for one- and two-piece systems, it will be noted.

- Remove appliance gently without pulling the wafer off.
- If using a two-piece system, remove the flange and pouch as one piece.
- Save the closure clip if using an open-end system.
- Dispose of the old appliance.
- Remove any excess stool or mucus around the stoma with a dry cloth.
- Gently clean stoma and surrounding skin.
- Follow pouch instructions about how much space to leave between the stoma and the skin barrier.
- Trace measurement on the back of the flange (two-piece system) or center (one-piece system).
- Cut opening and remove center backing paper.
- If using adhesive paste, apply to skin around stoma.
- Center the flange (two-piece system) or appliance (one-piece system) over the stoma.
- Remove the remaining backing paper.
- If using a two-piece system, secure pouch to flange.
- If using an open-end system, apply closure clip.

Hygiene

You can bathe normally with or without your pouching system in place. Be sure to avoid using soaps, scrubs, or creams on the area around the stoma (this may irritate the skin).

A Day in the Life

Many new ostomates worry that their procedure will interfere with their daily activities. However, most ostomates report *more* involvement in and enjoyment of daily activities now that they have less pain and don't have to worry about flare ups. In this section, we will discuss, briefly, the impact of ostomy surgery on diet, exercise, clothing, work/social life, sex/intimacy, and travel.

Diet

After an ostomy procedure has healed, you should return to a normal diet. Unless you have other medical issues in addition to an IBD, your diet will no longer be restricted.

There is one (yes, only one) dietary requirement for people with ostomies: chew your food thoroughly. Chewing food well ensures that it will not cause any clogs or blockages (we'll talk more about those later).

If you are worried about the effects of food on digestion (i.e. foods that tend to cause gas) here is a list of foods and the digestive processes they tend to affect. Keep in mind that people react to foods differently, so these foods may not affect you in the ways outlined below.

Foods that tend to cause gas:

- Asparagus
- Beans
- Beer
- Broccoli
- Brussels sprouts
- Cabbage
- Carbonated beverages
- Cauliflower
- Onions
- Peas

Foods that tend to cause incomplete digestion:

- Apple peels
- Cabbage
- Celery
- Coconut
- Corn
- Dried fruit
- Mushrooms
- Nuts
- Pineapple
- Popcorn
- Seeds
- Skins from fruits and vegetables

Foods that tend to cause thickened stool:

- Applesauce
- Bananas
- Cheese
- Pasta
- Rice
- Creamy peanut butter
- Potatoes (without skin)

Foods that tend to cause thinned stool:

- Fried food
- Grape juice
- High sugar foods
- Prune juice
- Spicy foods

Foods that tend to cause increased odor:

- Alcohol
- Asparagus
- Broccoli
- Dried beans
- Eggs
- Fish
- Garlic
- Onions
- Peas

Foods that tend to cause reduced odor:

- Buttermilk
- Cranberry juice
- Parsley
- Yogurt

Exercise/Sports

Athletically speaking, ostomates can do anything non-ostomates can, although it is advisable to speak to your doctor before resuming or beginning strenuous activities. Contact sports are not recommended, but special equipment can be purchased to make participation possible. Weight-lifting does carry some risks, but these can also be overcome by taking the proper precautions. Even swimming is possible, which is great because swimming is terrific exercise, although as discussed earlier, it can decrease the wear time of skin barriers. Special swim wraps can be purchased to minimize the "bulge" of the bag under a fitted swimsuit and to protect the wafer and bag from the water.

Clothing

Having a pouch doesn't mean you can't have style! Because of the location of ostomy pouches, they are easily unnoticed in many of today's fashions. For extra coverage, there are many options available for both men and women.

For both men and women, a variety of undergarments can be used to hide the pouch "bulge" and hold it in place. For men, an ostomy wrap may help but many men feel most comfortable in jockey shorts with a built-in support pocket for the pouch. For women, stretch underpants or panty hose can cover and secure a pouch, as can camisoles worn under shirts and dresses. You can wear fairly snug pants and even fitted skirts. There is no question that the "bulge" of a full pouch might be detectable through your clothes. But remember! Many women without ostomies bemoan the "bulge" of their tummies after a full meal. All that solid food and water has to go somewhere as it passes through your digestive tract. It's either going to be inside the skin of your abdomen or outside it, but it's there either way. Emptying your pouch somewhat more frequently might make you feel less self-conscious on days when you are wearing particularly fitted outfits.

Work/Social Life

If your job does not involve heavy lifting, there is absolutely nothing to prevent you from winning employee of the month once your recovery period has ended. If your job does involve heavy lifting, talk to your doctor.

Telling people about an ostomy is often difficult for new ostomates. Even people who have lived with an ostomy for a long time may not be comfortable discussing it. This is perfectly understandable. It's the most extreme example of the secrecy often practiced by people living with an IBD. But don't let shame keep you silent with people who care about you. Deciding who to tell about your ostomy should be on a need-to-know basis. If you don't think someone needs to know, they probably don't. The people in your life who do need to be informed tend to be the people who are affected by it (serious partners, potential serious partners, occasionally co-workers in certain situations, etc.). You can use your own discretion for who to tell and how much detail to divulge.

Many people find it helpful to rehearse a speech beforehand. Possible talking points include:

- The fact that you have a history of GI issues.
- The fact that you had abdominal surgery.
- The fact that you now use a device to collect waste.

   a   If you are speaking to a boss and/or coworker, this could be a good segue into any circumstances/limitations they may need to know about.

- The fact that you are okay and can now enjoy all the things you couldn't when you were sick.

As in revealing any sensitive matter, or even just the fact that you have an IBD, many, in fact most, people will be concerned for your well-being and curious about your condition. Allowing them to ask questions might make both of you more comfortable with the situation. However, if they ask a question that you feel is too personal or that you are unable or don't want to answer, you can tell them that there are a lot of wonderful resources on the web if they're interested in ostomy procedures. Be sure to speak about your ostomy in a positive way. If you view it positively, so will they!

Sex/Intimacy

When discussing sex, the most important thing to remember is that ostomy or not, there is *no* such thing as a "normal" sex life. Healthy, satisfying sexuality is as varied as the great cuisines of the world and people have personal tastes, preferences, likes and dislikes that are both individual and couple specific.

That being said, having an ostomy should not interfere with typical sexual intercourse. Close body contact and movement will not hurt the stoma, or dislodge the pouch. Neither penetration nor orgasm will injure the stoma of either a man or a woman. You should *not* use the stoma itself for sex, nor should you be on the receiving end of anal sex if you have an ostomy. But aside from these specific caveats, really nothing is off limits.

Deciding when to resume sexual activity after a procedure should depend on both your comfort level and your physical healing. A good rule of thumb is that if you can walk a half mile without losing your breath, you are physically capable of resuming intercourse. Emotionally, however, you may take more or less time to "heal." If you have a regular partner already, it might be helpful to start "small" with other intimate activities like masturbation. This can help you build confidence as well as put your fears about intimacy to rest. If you have a stable partner, he/she is probably already aware of your ostomy. It might be helpful to allow your partner to ask your ostomy nurse his/her own questions.

Telling a new partner about your ostomy can be scary, but it shouldn't get in the way of your dating life. Although rejection is always a possibility, you should probably find a way to raise the issue *before* you end up in the bedroom with someone. Indeed, one way to positively frame an ostomy is that it is a great *test* of any new partner. If they are considerate, understanding and sensitive about it, that speaks well of their character and their potential as a partner. If they are rude, insensitive or rejecting, trust me – you didn't want to partner with them anyway.

I have never had to live with ostomy. But I do have another issue that made dating feel pretty complicated. When I was 18 months old, I was badly burned when I pulled a boiling pot over on myself. I have significant burn scars on my neck, shoulders, upper arms, breasts and chest. When I was 13, I had skin graft surgery that transplanted a good bit of skin from my left thigh to "patches" on my chest near my shoulders and over my breasts. My upper body looks a bit like a mottled patchwork quilt, and the donor site on my thigh has bizarrely straight lined square and rectangular patches of thickened, puckered scar tissue as well. I can mostly cover my scars, even in summer, with short sleeve shirts and crew neck shirts. I never wear V-neck dresses or blouses as the "V" nicely frames a particularly mottled bit of grafted patchwork skin. But in most serious dating relationships, there came a point when the shirts came off and my scars were revealed in all their glory. I have often thought that if I had three wishes to squander selfishly (and not on, say, world peace), I would wish to not have the scars. It would be nice to shop for clothes without so many constraints, and to wear a bathing suit or a tank top without people staring, however surreptitiously or politely, at the skin on my chest and arms. But interestingly, I would definitely *not* wish to have *never* had my scars. Having scars makes you more empathic and more sensitive to the needs of others. It makes you know that what really counts about a person is what's on the inside, and that beauty is, truly, not about what's on the surface.

My scars were also a fantastic litmus test for boyfriends. One jerk I dated for a while in college told me, "By the way, I think your scars are disgusting," shortly after I broke up with him. That certainly confirmed my decision to dump him! I am happy to report that when I finally got the courage to *ask* a serious boyfriend what he thought – truly – about my scars, he replied, without missing a beat, "I think they make you interesting." Sensibly, I married him. Thirty years later I still think it was probably the best decision I ever made. People who love you will think you're attractive no matter what. It's important to remember that.

Deciding when to tell a romantic interest about your ostomy is totally up to you. There's no right or wrong time to tell someone, although it is probably advisable to tell a partner before sexual activity occurs to avoid awkward questions and surprises. Some people prefer to tell new partners early on in the relationship so that if the partner isn't comfortable with the ostomy, it's less disappointing since there was less at stake. Other people prefer to wait until the partner gets to know them so the partner can make a better-informed decision. Just like telling a boss or friend, it might be easier to rehearse a speech about what you want to say to a current/potential partner.

There are some tips for making sexual intercourse more comfortable for you and your partner. Keeping bags covered and held in place can make you feel more at ease and create a wider range of motion. To do this, women can wear ostomy lingerie, a tube top over the bottom half of the abdomen, or crotchless underwear and men can wear shorts with openings or a specially designed wrap around the middle.

Although sexual function should return normally, some people do experience problems, particularly immediately following the procedure. Some men report difficulty attaining or maintaining an erection in the immediate post-op period. If this is related to the surgery, it will subside fairly soon afterwards. If dysfunction persists, it may be psychological. There's nothing quite like performance anxiety to kill arousal for most guys. If you get too up in your head, it gets very difficult to enjoy the sensations of the moment. Often, there is a vicious cycle of dysfunction during intercourse leading to negative self-evaluations and low expectations, which in turn cause impotence in another sexual encounter, and so on. If impotence is not going away after the immediate post-op period, try to think of alternative explanations (the vicious cycle above, attempting intercourse when exhausted, etc.). It could be helpful to talk to a medical and/or mental health professional to determine potential causes and solutions.

Women with ileostomies need to be especially careful with birth control methods. Because birth control pills are often absorbed in the lining of the intestine, the procedure may interfere with their function. Talk to your doctor about alternative birth control methods. For women, there are three potential (though unlikely) sexual issues that can result from an ostomy: tenderness in the perineal wound (area where rectum is removed) for a certain post-op period, which can make intercourse uncomfortable, the uterus taking over the space where the colon originally was located, which can cause discomfort during intercourse, decreased sensitivity of the clitoris, and vaginal dryness. If you are experiencing any of these problems, you can use this as an excuse to start experimenting with different positions. Also, lubricant can be very helpful. If you are still experiencing discomfort, speak to a medical professional about possible solutions.

Travel

Traveling with an ostomy is totally fine, although it is advisable to bring double the amount of supplies you think you need (better safe than sorry). When checking baggage, it is also a good idea to split supplies between checked bags and carry-on bags in case your checked luggage gets misplaced. If you're taking a road trip, store supplies in the coolest part of the car and avoid the trunk and back window ledge.

Common Concerns

Leakage

Shit happens, literally. Unfortunately, leakages do happen, although they are almost always preventable. The majority of ostomates blame leakages on personal mistakes such as not checking to make sure the clip or seal on their pouch is tight enough, using a new pouching system to which they haven't adjusted, or having a pouch system that is not compatible with their particular stoma shape and/or size.

The main solution is to be proactive. Be careful and methodical when applying and sealing a new pouch. If you're ordering a new pouch system, do a "trial run" while you finish out the supply of your old system: you can wear the new system at times you're not planning to leave the house and see how you adjust.

Many ostomates report issues with night leakages. To avoid this, use appliances with larger bags/pouches for nighttime hours and, if using an open-end system, drain before bed.

Like fecal incontinence, people are often terrified of leakage. The key to surviving without being overwhelmed by worry is to remind yourself that even if your pouch does leak, it is *not* a catastrophe. Inconvenient? Absolutely. A bit embarrassing? Certainly. But you know how to clean up. If you are experimenting with a new system, keep a change of clothes in your car or stashed at work.

Blockages

Sometimes, stool can accumulate and plug up the bowel, causing a blockage. This is more likely to occur in people with ileostomies, although colostomy patients can have blockages too. When you have a blockage, your stoma will be inactive or output will be unusually watery. To try to loosen up the stool, you can try taking a warm bath to relax abdominal muscles, getting on the floor in a knee to chest position, or massaging the area around the stoma. If your stoma is inactive for four to six hours, accompanied by cramping or nausea, call your doctor. To avoid blockages, make sure to chew your food well, especially when eating high residue foods such as pineapple, nuts, coconut, celery and corn.

Catastrophic Thoughts

As you know, catastrophic thoughts can occur about lots of different things in lots of different situations for everyone, IBD or not. Catastrophic thoughts about ostomies may seem particularly scary and plausible. But a little consideration of the evidence may put many of your fears to rest. For example, you may think that *everyone* notices your ostomy bag under your clothing. But do they really? Let's look at the evidence. According to a UOAA (United Ostomy Associations of America), 1.5–2 million people have ostomies. That's a lot of folks out there! Early on in my career I had a client with an ostomy and I had *no idea* until his wife told me. (They were actually in treatment to help her manage her obsessive-compulsive disorder, and its impact on the family, and not specifically for him.) So, chances are you've come across at least one ostomate and *never noticed*.

You also may think that everyone hears that gurgle from your stoma or the release of gas. Don't forget that even people without ostomies or IBDs make the occasional stomach grumble or gas bubble. Most likely if someone even notices your noises or gas, they'll attribute it to an everyday phenomenon or to someone else.

You may well think that your ostomy is ugly or that your stoma is disgusting in some way. You might be surprised by how invisible it is to others, even if they're looking right at it. You might even be surprised by the degree to which people who love you see your ostomy as *part* of the "you" they love. When my daughter was 11, she called my scars my "lacy skin" and told me she thinks they're pretty. In the eyes of love, even stomas can look like dimples.

Your ostomy may well have saved your life. If you love it, everyone around you will too.

Find Out More

For more tips and information about new products check out the various ostomy message boards, the UOAA website, and the UOAA's quarterly magazine called *The Phoenix*.

11 Summary and Review

I started out by reviewing differential diagnosis and considering other conditions that might look like an IBD based on symptoms, or might actually be co-morbid with an IBD (meaning you can have both disorders at the same time). Having an IBD actually puts you at somewhat greater than normal risk for having celiac disease (meaning you can't tolerate gluten), and during active flares some people with IBDs are more likely to show evidence of lactose intolerance, so you should definitely be evaluated for both. But food intolerance doesn't *explain* IBD and if you're not actually gluten or lactose intolerant, there's no reason to limit those foods.

Many people with an IBD were misdiagnosed (sometimes for years!) with IBS, so it can be very frustrating to hear a doctor say that your IBD is in remission, but you're still having symptoms because *now* you have secondary IBS. Unfortunately, it *is* possible to have both an inflammatory bowel disease and symptoms that are consistent with a centralized pain processing disorder like IBS, especially if you continue to have significant GI symptoms when the IBD is in remission. IBD and IBS may share some underlying biology (like inflammation and disruption in the normal eco-system of intestinal bacteria) and also share things like visceral hypersensitivity. So learning to tell the difference between abdominal pain that signals a return of an IBD flare and gut discomfort that may simply be consistent with IBS is an important part of learning to manage your condition.

I also reviewed some of the theories about what causes IBDs – almost certainly a combination of genetics, living in weirdly sterile environments (which results in increased autoimmune disorders in western industrial societies) and possibly overuse of antibiotics, all of which can lead to disruptions in the human microbiome in the gut and inflammatory processes in which the immune system starts attacking both good bacteria and gut tissue itself.

It's important to remember that stress can definitely contribute to the inflammatory process, but it doesn't *cause* it. That is, your IBD is in no way your fault. But you might be able to influence the course of the disorder by engaging in effective stress management. Stress has a physical effect on the gut for everyone, no matter what else is going on biologically, so managing stress effectively should help reduce your GI symptoms no matter what. And gut

DOI: 10.4324/9781003057635-12

problems are stressful, no matter what caused them to begin with. Even a Buddhist monk who spends four hours a day meditating might still have an active IBD, and you might find that you remain in remission even during times of notable stress. Still, in so far as stress contributes to inflammation, and because feeling stressed out is miserable no matter what else is going on, learning effective relaxation and stress management strategies can only help, and certainly can't hurt.

So, I strongly suggested that you regularly practice one or more relaxation techniques. Since the physiological arousal associated with stress can actually make GI symptoms worse, reducing physiological arousal can be very helpful. Deep breathing, done correctly, is a particularly useful exercise because it can be done anywhere, any time, without anyone noticing. It will reduce heart rate and blood pressure, suppress the release of stress hormones, and can help optimize intestinal motility. Even if imagery and/or progressive muscle relaxation work well for you – and it's great if they do – I do suggest that you keep working on deep breathing until you can feel yourself relax after two to three deep breaths.

I then introduced the basic cognitive model, which suggests that our reactions to situations – our feelings, physical symptoms and behaviors – are the result of our *beliefs* about situations, rather than the situations themselves. Oftentimes, people with gut problems have lots of negative beliefs. Some of those negative beliefs are general ones that occur across lots of different types of situations. Some of those negative beliefs relate directly to GI symptoms themselves. GI-related beliefs tend to fall into two categories: beliefs about how intolerable symptoms are and beliefs about the social and occupational implications of symptoms. Since beliefs can be right or wrong, it makes a lot of sense to identify our negative thoughts and try to look at them a bit more objectively. This includes trying to generate *benign alternatives* to our negative beliefs, and then considering the evidence we have for and against each set of beliefs. *Behavioral experiments*, which can provide us with relevant data we wouldn't normally have access to, can be very helpful in challenging deeply held or upsetting beliefs.

The best way to learn these techniques is to practice them, usually by actually writing up a worksheet, after the fact, when you have a little more distance and perspective, and can take the time to think things through. Eventually, though, it would be much more useful to you if you could begin to identify and question your negative automatic thoughts *in the moment*, while stressful things are actually occurring. Now obviously you can't just whip out a worksheet during a meeting or while you're on a date or talking to your kid's teacher. That *would* be weird! But the nice thing about this is that the more you practice coming up with benign alternatives to negative thoughts, the more automatic *positive* thoughts will start to become. Most people find that they don't need to keep using the actual worksheets for very long. They begin to catch the negative thoughts right as they crop up. Eventually, you start to question those thoughts the instant they occur to you. People report thoughts like this:

Oh God, my gut is acting up and I'm going to have to step out of the meeting. My boss is going to think I'm an idiot. This is going to be awful. Wait a second – that's probably not true. I did a good job preparing the report... if I have to step out for a few minutes I can just finish the discussion when I get back. My gut is acting up, but that can't stop me from finishing this...

When I see people in my private practice, they often tell me that at first the positive thoughts actually sound like they're in my voice! People will tell me they hear me saying to them, "Now wait a second... is that the most accurate way of thinking about it? What's the evidence?" We usually have a good laugh about it – they can't get rid of me! Eventually, though, as people get better at it, the positive thoughts start to be in their own voice. By the end of treatment, they're often not even conscious of the process of questioning negative thoughts and replacing them with more reasonable ones. It just starts to happen automatically. Negative thoughts still occur to them from time to time, but they have much less power, and feel much less compelling and upsetting. People are able to dismiss them much more quickly.

Because this book doesn't take long to work through, you may not find that this happens to you right away. It may take weeks or even several more months. Don't give up! Keep practicing things after the fact, and eventually you'll start to be able to do it in the moment, when stressful things are actually happening. Even if you can't do it in the moment, lots of times we ruminate and obsess about upsetting things after the fact. If these skills help you do less of that, then that's a good thing too.

The final piece of any treatment program for gut related problems involves identifying situations that people have been *avoiding*, including examples of *subtle avoidance*, and then using the techniques of exposure therapy to try to overcome that avoidance. Avoidance is often the most life-damaging aspect of GI problems – more than any physical discomfort or inconvenience. Many people with an IBD experience a great deal of *shame* about their disease and work very hard to keep their condition *secret* – avoiding telling people why they can't eat out or may need more frequent bathroom breaks. This contributes to avoidance of intimacy and often deprives you of the opportunity to get support and understanding and to structure your work and personal life in ways that allow you to function optimally. People with IBDs often try to avoid *eating* during the day to minimize discomfort and the inconvenience of frequent bathroom visits. Fasting during the day is *not* a great strategy for people who are already having difficulty maintaining their weight and getting adequate nutrition. Sometimes avoidance gets so bad that people stop traveling, stop eating out, stop going to parties, stop shopping, sometimes even stop working and socializing all together. If this is you, you've allowed your gut problems to cheat you out of work, love and play – the three most essential components of any healthy, happy life. It's essential that you take your life back. Don't allow negative, catastrophic thoughts that may not even be true to limit what you do or where you go. Use the techniques outlined in Chapter 7 on eliminating avoidance – reread the chapter if you need to – to help you design an individualized program that will get you back to all aspects of living.

In Chapter 8 I reviewed what's known about diet and nutrition in IBDs. There are really two different things to worry about – managing active flares and getting adequate nutrition overall. When you are in an active flare, especially if you have strictures or have a history of small bowel obstructions, it is very important to follow your doctor's advice about limiting high residue foods. Your doctor (and medical nutritionist) will almost certainly counsel you to limit or completely avoid insoluble fiber (found in wheat and corn bran, fruit and vegetable skins and certain hard seeds and kernels) and various high residue foods like popcorn, nuts, seeds, skins and stringy or fibrous foods like celery. When you are *not* in flare, eating a healthful, balanced diet that combines plenty of soluble fiber (found in rice and oats, legumes and the flesh of many fruits and vegetables) with plenty of protein (from meat, dairy, eggs, fish or legumes combined with rice) and as wide a variety of fresh, natural foods as you can is the best way to maximize nutrition and overall health. There is *no* universal "IBD" diet and eating the *least* restrictive diet possible is the best way to nourish your body and keep you healthy and vital. The low FODMAP diet does lead to a reduction in symptoms for many IBD patients, and can be used short term to get some relief and help your gut calm down. But! It's incredibly restrictive, and not a good option for long term nutrition, a healthy microbiome and a reasonable social life. If you find from experience that you truly must limit or eliminate certain foods, be sure to replace them with nutritionally equivalent foods. With your doctor's advice, you might also consider supplementing with pro-biotics or certain vitamins (like D or B12) to replenish your microbiome and replace lost nutrients that your gut doesn't absorb well. In the end, the important thing is not to *fear* food or fall prey to the fanatics who insist that there is a magic IBD diet that will cure you if only you always avoid gluten or dairy or soy or meat or eggs or fructose or sorbitol or alcohol or fiber or carbohydrates or fat or all of the above. In the end, eating a healthful, varied, natural foods diet is by far the best way to manage both inflammation and nutrition.

Medical management of an IBD can be complicated and anxiety provoking, and often raises difficult decisions about balancing the relative risks and benefits of pursuing different treatment options AND of not pursuing those options. In Chapter 9 I reviewed a number of aspects of medical management, including the doctor/patient relationship; scopes and other diagnostic techniques; steroids, which most IBD patients have a love/hate relationship with; other medication options; and surgery. Your doctor is the expert in this area – but you should always view yourself as an essential member of your own treatment team. Different people prefer different levels of information. Some people really like to know all the ins and outs of how each treatment option works so that they can make as informed a decision as possible about their own care. Other people strongly prefer the doctor to just make a recommendation. They're the one who went to medical school, after all! Either strategy is fine if it works well and feels comfortable for you. But you should always know enough to keep yourself from catastrophizing and to make decisions based on actual risks. For example, while it might be true that a particular medication is potentially dangerous for your liver, you can be assured that your doctor would never let it get to that point, because he or she would monitor your liver's health with regular blood tests and would take you off the medication if there were signs that your liver was reacting badly. While it's true that some IBD medications increase your risk of certain cancers, remember that an unmanaged IBD can increase your risk of *other* cancers. So don't let fear be the only thing that affects your decisions. You should also know enough to be an accurate reporter back to your doctor about the effects and any possible side effects of a medication you're taking. Don't ever worry about *bothering* your doctor. They won't be annoyed with you for informing them about a new side effect, reaction or experience. They will appreciate you taking a proactive role in managing your own care. Doctors hate being in the dark, and you are the only one who can let them know what's actually going on with you.

In Chapter 10 we talked about the possibility many people with an IBD fear the most – the need for an ostomy. There is no doubt that ostomies are the treatment of last resort, and that they are complicated to adjust to and to manage. But the reality is that most people with ostomies are so relieved to be out of pain, and to be able to eat pretty much whatever they want whenever they want, that they are able to be far more active and involved with life than they were before they got the ostomy. Using humor, including loved ones and close coworkers in your circle of intimacy, and combating catastrophic thoughts related to your ostomy with evidence and benign alternatives will all go a long way to helping you adjust successfully. As with every other aspect of managing your IBD, and life in general, don't fall prey to shame, to avoidance or to negative, catastrophic distortions about what other people will see or think or how they will react.

As a final exercise, it might be interesting to revisit the questionnaires you completed at the beginning of the book – the ones that measured visceral sensitivity and catastrophic beliefs about GI symptoms and fear of food. You can find them again now in Appendices A, B and C. Try filling them out again with a different color pen. Most people will find that their scores have changed a lot. If that's you, congratulations! You are well on your way to reclaiming your life from your inflammatory bowel disorder.

When to Ask for Professional Help

I really hope this book has been helpful to you and that you feel better able to cope with your IBD than before you worked through this program. However, it's important to acknowledge that not everyone will be able to get everything they need from a self-help book. Sometimes problems are just too complicated, long-standing or more entrenched. Many people with IBDs also face other challenges. People with an IBD are somewhat more likely than people in general to struggle with depression and anxiety, mostly because having an IBD can be really stressful. Self-help is great, but there's nothing quite like having a dedicated, supportive, and highly skilled professional working with you to understand and address the places where you're getting stuck. If you feel like you're still struggling – if you're unhappy, unmotivated, exhausted, over-whelmed, or worried a lot of the time, or if you feel like your gut symptoms are still impairing your quality of life, then it may be time to think about seeking professional help from a psychiatrist or a psychologist with a back-ground in *cognitive-behavioral therapy*.

Almost all therapists (including social workers, counselors, psychologists, and psychiatrists) are warm, caring, supportive people. They wouldn't have gone into the field if they weren't. But not all therapists are trained the same way. Some therapists may be very kind and personally insightful, but may not have the specific skills they need to help with particular problems. Cognitive-behavioral therapy (CBT) is one of the few types of therapy that has been proven to work for a wide range of problems, including depression, panic disorder, social anxiety disorder, generalized anxiety disorder, obsessive-compulsive disorder, and a range of chronic health-related issues. A good way to find out if there is a CBT therapist close to you is to visit the Find a Therapist webpages at one of the professional organizations that specializes in promoting good science in the diagnosis and treatment of behavioral health concerns. These organizations include the Association of Behavioral and Cognitive Therapies (ABCT.org), the Anxiety and Depression Association of America (ADAA.org), and the Academy of Cognitive and Behavioral Therapies (academyofct.org). All three websites allow you to search geographically to find therapists in your area. One silver lining of the COVID pandemic is that most therapists are now able to see people securely via telehealth. As long as you live in a state in which the therapist is licensed, you may well be able to see them even if you live hundreds of miles away. If you can't find someone in your state, try calling your insurance provider and asking specifically if the company has any therapists in its network who are trained in CBT.

One final option to consider is medication – not another round of ster-oids – but medications that work in the brain to help modulate the neu-rochemicals involved in depression, anxiety, and pain. You will typically need to see a psychiatrist for this (although some internists, general practi-tioners, and gastroenterologists might feel comfortable and confident pre-scribing these particular medicines for the treatment of someone with an IBD). The neuromodulators with a good scientific track record in helping people with various physical health problems are several different groups of medicines collectively known as "antidepressants." The name is misleading, because many medicines can be used to treat different things. For example, aspirin can be used to reduce fever. It can also be used to reduce the pain of migraine headaches and the very different pain of sore muscles. It can *also* be used to reduce the risk of having a heart attack or stroke, because it affects the development of blood clots. So if we called aspirin an "anti-fever" drug, it really wouldn't tell the whole story and it would be confusing. Why would I take an anti-fever drug to reduce my risk of heart attack? Because of course aspirin isn't *just* an anti-fever drug. The same thing is true of the so-called antidepressants. These medicines aren't *just* antidepressants. They can affect a number of different processes, including digestion and pain.

There are three basic classes of neuromodulators that might make sense to consider. The oldest group is known as the tricyclic family (TCAs). They mostly affect a neurotransmitter in the brain called norepinephrine. They've been around for decades and they're all available generically (so they're less expensive). TCAs include:

- Amitriptyline (Elavil)
- Imipramine (Tofranil)
- Desipramine (Norpramin)
- Nortriptyline (Pamelor)

TCAs tend to cause "constipation" as a side effect. This might be pretty inconvenient for someone who was taking the medicine for depression, but for someone with an IBD who suffers from chronic diarrhea, this can be a terrific outcome that can help normalize bowel movements. One study found that TCAs could be quite helpful in managing residual symptoms of an IBD in people who were on appropriate medical therapy.[1]

The next family of medicines is the selective serotonin reuptake inhibitors (SSRIs). The first, and most famous, SSRI was Prozac (Fluoxetine), but there are many others, including:

- Sertraline (Zoloft)
- Citalopram (Celexa)
- Escitalopram (Lexapro)
- Paroxetine (Paxil)

SSRIs tend to cause diarrhea, at least initially, when people start taking them, so they are better to use when your disease is in remission or is only mild. They can help a lot with stress reactivity, depression and anxiety, though, so if the SSRI-driven exacerbation of diarrhea resolves relatively quickly, they can be pretty helpful.

The final and newest family of medicines are those called serotonin-norepinephrine reuptake inhibitors (SNRIs). They include:

- Venlafaxine (Effexor)
- Duloxetine (Cymbalta)
- Desvenlavaxine (Pristiq)
- Milnacipram (Savella)

Interestingly, the SNRIs have been found to be quite helpful in treating chronic pain conditions, like fibromyalgia and peripheral neuropathy, and some preliminary studies have suggested they help with visceral (gut) pain as well.[2] Because they affect both norepinephrine (which can make you constipated) and serotonin (which can give you diarrhea), the GI side effects tend to cancel each other out and you mostly get the benefits of the anti-pain, anti-inflammatory (and antidepressant) effects, so the SNRIs may be especially helpful for people with IBDs.

It's important to understand that none of these medicines are "addictive" and you won't become "dependent" on them. There *are* medicines that are addictive and cause physiological dependence and tolerance – these include the stimulants (like Ritalin [methylphenidate] and Adderall [amphetamine and dextroamphetamine]) and the anti-anxiety drugs from the family called benzodiazepines (like Xanax [alprazolam], Valium [diazepam], and Klonopin [clonazepam]). Interestingly, all of these drugs are also sold illegally as "street drugs" because you can get high by taking them. No one would ever sell Elavil, Prozac, or Effexor illegally – because no one would buy it! You can't get "high" by taking them. They don't even elevate your mood. If you're depressed, they take at least two weeks (and often up to six weeks) to kick in and start making you feel better. They don't change your personality – although they can make negative, catastrophic thoughts less intense, and they might make it easier to learn and use the cognitive-therapy skills taught in this book. The relief you get from them isn't "fake" – it's just you at your best. If IBD patients find that a medicine is helping, most will elect to stay on it for at least six months to a year. Many people can go off at that point. Especially if you've worked through a program like this, you may well find that you don't need it anymore. On the other hand, if you find that you feel more depressed or anxious, or just that it's taking too much energy to manage your thoughts and feelings when you go off the medicine, then it might make a lot of sense to stay on the medication longer. This isn't a personal failure or a defeat. It's just smart, proactive management of a set of truly complex medical conditions.

Final Thoughts

It has been my privilege over the years to work with a number of incredibly brave, insightful patients who have suffered from a variety of health problems including serious GI disorders. I truly believe that an active, open, curious approach to life is the best one. You can learn to reduce physiological arousal (and inflammation) by practicing relaxation strategies. You can identify your own thoughts and core beliefs and learn to examine them more objectively. You can test your beliefs against your experiences in the world and take new evidence into account. You can courageously, with humor and clear matter-of-fact information let people in your life know about your IBD and what you need to do to manage it. You can bravely stop avoiding things and engage in meaningful work, love and play fully and joyfully. You can manage your disease proactively with your medical team.

None of these things will guarantee remission of your IBD. That is never entirely in our control. But they *will* allow you to reclaim your *life* and to *cope* with Crohn's and colitis as effectively as possible. And in the end, that's what matters most.

Notes

1 Iskander, H.N., Cassell, B., Kanuri, N., Gyawali, C.P., Gutierrez, A., Dassopoulos, T. & Sayuk, G.S. (2014). Tricylcic antidepressants for management of residual symptoms in inflammatory bowel disease. *Journal of Clinical Gastroenterology*, 48(5), 423–429.
2 Drossman, D.A. (2008). Severe and refractory chronic abdominal pain: treatment strategies. *Clinical Gastroenterology and Hepatology*, 6(9), 978–982.

Appendix A – Visceral Sensitivity Index (VSI)

Below are statements that describe how some people respond to symptoms or discomfort in their belly or lower abdomen. These may include pain, diarrhea, constipation, bloating or sense of urgency. Please answer *how strongly you agree or disagree* with each of these statements, AS THEY RELATE TO YOU. Answer all of the statements as honestly and thoughtfully as you can.

Item	Strongly disagree	Moder-ately disagree	Mildly disagree	Mildly agree	Moder-ately agree	Strongly agree
I worry that whenever I eat during the day, bloating and distension in my belly will get worse.	0	1	2	3	4	5
I get anxious when I go to a new restaurant.	0	1	2	3	4	5
I often worry about problems in my belly.	0	1	2	3	4	5
I have a difficult time enjoying myself because I cannot get my mind off of discomfort in my belly.	0	1	2	3	4	5
I often fear that I won't be able to have a normal bowel movement.	0	1	2	3	4	5
Because of fear of developing abdominal discomfort, I seldom try new foods.	0	1	2	3	4	5

DOI: 10.4324/9781003057635-13

Item	Strongly disagree	Moder- ately disagree	Mildly disagree	Mildly agree	Moder- ately agree	Strongly agree
No matter what I eat, I will probably feel uncomfortable.	0	1	2	3	4	5
As soon as I feel abdominal discomfort I begin to worry and feel anxious.	0	1	2	3	4	5
When I enter a place I haven't been before, one of the first things I do is to look for a bathroom.	0	1	2	3	4	5
I am constantly aware of the feelings I have in my belly.	0	1	2	3	4	5
I often feel discomfort in my belly could be a sign of a serious illness.	0	1	2	3	4	5
As soon as I awake, I worry that I will have discomfort in my belly during the day.	0	1	2	3	4	5
When I feel dis- comfort in my belly, it frightens me.	0	1	2	3	4	5
In stressful situations, my belly bothers me a lot.	0	1	2	3	4	5
I constantly think about what is hap- pening inside my belly.	0	1	2	3	4	5

To score the VSI, just add up the numbers you circled.   My score _____

Mild: 0–10
Moderate: 11–30
Severe: 31–75

Labus, J., Bolus, R., Chang, L., Wiklund, I., Naesdal, J., Mayer, E.A. & Naliboff, B.D. (2004). The Visceral Sensitivity Index: development and validation of a gastrointestinal symptom-specific anxiety scale. *Alimentary Pharmacology and Therapeutics, 20*, 89–97. Labus, J. (2007). The central role of gastrointestinal-specific anxiety in IBS: Further validation of the visceral sensitivity index. *Psychosomatic Medicine, 69*, 89–98.

Appendix B – GI Cognitions Questionnaire (GI-COG)

Please rate the degree to which you believe each of the following statements:

Item	Hardly at all	A little bit	Moder- ately	A fair bit	Very much
If I feel the urge to defecate and cannot find a bathroom right away I won't be able to hold it and I'll be incontinent.	0	1	2	3	4
The thought of fecal incontinence is terrifying. If it happened, I would never get over the humiliation.	0	1	2	3	4
If I fart, people around me will be disgusted.	0	1	2	3	4
If I don't drink or eat with other people, they will think I'm anti-social and no fun.	0	1	2	3	4
If I have to get up and leave an event, meeting or social gathering, to go to the bathroom people will think there's something wrong with me.	0	1	2	3	4
If I have to interrupt a meeting or presentation at work to go to the bathroom, it will be awful, and people will think I'm incompetent or unreliable.	0	1	2	3	4
If I have stop or leave to find a bathroom during an outing or trip, my friends and family will be frustrated and annoyed with me.	0	1	2	3	4
If I told my coworkers about my gut problems they wouldn't understand and would think I was weak or gross.	0	1	2	3	4

DOI: 10.4324/9781003057635-14

Item	Hardly at all	A little bit	Moder- ately	A fair bit	Very much
When I feel my GI symptoms acting up, I'm afraid the pain will be excruciating and intolerable.	0	1	2	3	4
When my gut acts up, I have to cancel my plans and miss out on important parts of life.	0	1	2	3	4
If I'm experiencing a gut attack and feeling sick, I can't enjoy or pay attention to anything else.	0	1	2	3	4
It is unfair and horrible that I have to have these awful symptoms.	0	1	2	3	4
If people knew about my gut pro- blems, they would think about me negatively.	0	1	2	3	4
If I leave the house without my emergency medicine(s) (e.g. Imo- dium, Lomotil, Pepto-Bismol, Gas-Ex, Tums) it could lead to disaster.	0	1	2	3	4
Having to deal with gut problems is incredibly embarrassing.	0	1	2	3	4
If people knew what my life was really like, they would think I was crazy.	0	1	2	3	4

To score the GI-COG, just add up the numbers you circled My score_____

Mild: 0–19
Moderate: 20–39
Severe: 40–64

Appendix C – Fear of Food Questionnaire (FFQ)

Please rate the degree to which you believe each of the following statements:

Item	Not at all	A little	Some-what	Moder-ately	Quite a bit	Abso-lutely
1. I try hard to identify foods that trigger GI symptoms.	0	1	2	3	4	5
2. I cannot tolerate certain foods.	0	1	2	3	4	5
3. I try to avoid eating trigger foods.	0	1	2	3	4	5
4. The range of foods it feels "safe" to eat has grown pretty narrow.	0	1	2	3	4	5
5. Sometimes I don't eat in order to avoid dealing with GI symptoms.	0	1	2	3	4	5
6. If I could survive without eating, it would be a huge relief.	0	1	2	3	4	5
7. I'm afraid of experiencing GI symptoms when I eat.	0	1	2	3	4	5
8. I'm afraid to eat certain foods.	0	1	2	3	4	5
9. Food sometimes feels like the enemy.	0	1	2	3	4	5
10. If a certain food triggers GI symptoms, I worry about eating it again.	0	1	2	3	4	5
11. I have lost too much weight because I avoid eating.	0	1	2	3	4	5
12. My restricted diet makes it harder to go out and socialize.	0	1	2	3	4	5

DOI: 10.4324/9781003057635-15

Item	Not at all	A little	Some-what	Moder-ately	Quite a bit	Abso-lutely
13. People in my life don't always support my efforts to eliminate trigger foods from my diet.	0	1	2	3	4	5
14. My restricted diet some-times causes conflict with people in my life.	0	1	2	3	4	5
15. I can't enjoy food the way I used to.	0	1	2	3	4	5
16. I have had to give up foods that I enjoy.	0	1	2	3	4	5
17. I really miss eating certain foods.	0	1	2	3	4	5
18. My restrictive diet frustrates me.	0	1	2	3	4	5

To score the FFQ, just add up the numbers you circled: My score_____

None: 0–15
Mild: 16–30
Moderate: 31–45
Severe: 46–90

Appendix D – Sample Treatment Protocols

This appendix contains two sample treatment protocols for the cases presented at the beginning of the book. Both cases are hypothetical, but are based loosely on compilations of a number of real patients treated by the author.

For patients, if you are wondering if working with a cognitive-behavioral therapist might be right for you, reading these cases might give you a sense of what that could look like. You might or might not "see" yourself in either case, but the general approach of the therapist should be similar if you were to seek out therapy yourself.

If you are a therapist or counselor who is working with patients with IBD, these treatment protocols are illustrative examples of two very different kinds of cases. While the two cases differ considerably in many details (age and sex of patient, severity and type of IBD, presence of secondary IBS, psychiatric co-morbidity, and so on) there are also parallels, and both treatment protocols follow a recognizable arc. If you are experienced in CBT more generally, reading through these treatment protocols should give you a good idea of how to apply CBT specifically to patients with an IBD. If you are less familiar with CBT principles and approaches, I hope these case summaries will help you appreciate both the power and the flexibility and scope of the approach. CBT is often caricatured as a collection of "techniques" that ignores the therapeutic relationship, and doesn't pay attention to the patient's history or their current context and family system. Nothing could be further from the truth. CBT is a comprehensive system of psychotherapy that takes into account early development, family history, and current context and functioning. Moreover, there is no way a patient will share their deepest fears and darkest secrets with you if haven't established a trusting therapeutic relationship, and they certainly won't be willing to take risks in therapy (like exposure therapy) if they don't trust the therapist's expertise, compassion and care. My hope is that these case examples will both inform and inspire your care for these patients.

If you are a gastroenterologist, nurse specialist or nurse practitioner in gastroenterology, I hope that these examples will illustrate how collaborating with a good CBT therapist can enhance your ability to work with patients successfully. Note that in both cases, the therapist urges the patient to be compliant with medication, to be honest and forthcoming with their doctor, to trust their

DOI: 10.4324/9781003057635-16

doctor's medical advice, and to collaborate actively in their own care. In both cases, the therapy enhanced the efficacy of the medical care, and resulted in better outcomes and more satisfied patients (and probably less stressed doctors as well!).

Case 1: Susannah

Session 1

Recall that Susannah, the young elementary school teacher in training, has just recently been diagnosed with ulcerative colitis. She is feeling overwhelmed and hopeless, and really wonders if she will be able to continue in her career (which she loves) or to make a life with her fiancé (whom she adores). She has lost weight and has been feeling so fatigued, sore and ill that she has stopped exercising. It is all she can do to show up for her courses and her student teaching. In the first session, a CBT therapist takes a thorough history, including eliciting information about family of origin, social and academic development, and history of psychiatric symptoms and diagnoses in her family and in Susannah herself. She has always been a happy, healthy, well-adjusted individual, but she is currently experiencing a number of symptoms of depression that don't quite meet criteria for a major depressive disorder. She is also anxious and overwhelmed about all the decisions she feels she has to make. She's having difficulty getting to sleep at night because she lies in bed with her thoughts racing. In light of all this, the best diagnosis appears to be an Adjustment Disorder with mixed Anxious and Depressed Mood. Indeed, the very fact that she has always been so healthy seems to be a risk factor for adjustment at the moment. Apart from the normal coughs, colds and occasional stomach bugs of childhood and adolescence, and a serious sprained ankle when she was playing competitive soccer in high school, Susannah has never really had to deal with serious medical issues before. She is convinced that this diagnosis spells the end of all her hopes and plans for a fulfilling life, and it makes her feel quite panicky when she thinks about it.

The therapist secures Susannah's consent to consult with the gastro-enterologist to ensure that the therapist is fully informed about the extent of Susannah's illness and the steps the gastroenterologist plans to take to manage it. Susannah is actually quite grateful that the therapist is willing to do this. She wants someone else to help her navigate the complexities of this, and she admits that she tends to feel intimidated when talking to her doctor and can't even think of what questions to ask as she tries to absorb what the doctor is saying.

Next, the therapist does some basic psychoeducation, and assures Susannah that the vast majority of UC patients live full, rich lives, and that there is no need to give up on her hopes and dreams. Susannah expresses relief at this, although she is still uncertain how she's going to cope with the physical challenges and the treatment protocols. She has never liked taking medication –

not even Tylenol – and is very reluctant to fill the prescription for mesalamine that the gastroenterologist gave her. The therapist talks through some of her concerns, and points out that the medication acts primarily in the colon to reduce inflammation, and that it should begin to provide her some symptomatic relief relatively quickly, and will allow the tissues in her gut to start healing. In fact, it has a good chance of inducing remission. Susannah raises concerns about the possibility of having to stay on the drug if she ever wanted to get pregnant. The therapist smiles and points out how quickly her perspective has shifted. When she started the session, she seemed convinced that she would never be able to marry, and now she's worrying about getting pregnant! Susannah also smiles, and admits that she is already feeling less anxious knowing that someone will be with her to walk her through this journey.

The therapist then explains how anxiety exacerbates some of the physical symptoms Susannah experiences through sympathetic nervous system arousal and assures Susannah that although these sensations are extremely uncomfortable, they are not dangerous. In fact, it is the body reacting normatively to a perceived threat. If the threat were a saber-toothed tiger, the body's "panicky" reaction (increasing respiration and heart rate, secreting adrenaline and cortisol, converting glycogen to glucose, and shutting down digestion) would be quite adaptive! The therapist then teaches Susannah deep diaphragmatic breathing to show her that she has some control over sympathetic versus parasympathetic arousal. Susannah likes this exercise. Although she has recently felt like her body was betraying her, as a former athlete she has always enjoyed practicing physical skills, and she gets the hang of it pretty quickly.

The therapist also reviews some basic insomnia management strategies. Like most people, when she can't sleep, Susannah stays in bed thinking it is better to at least "rest" even if she can't sleep. She is surprised when the therapist tells her this is a terrible idea! The therapist explains that staying in bed when you're anxious and frustrated about not being able to sleep just ends up creating an association between bed and anxious arousal – the opposite of what you need to fall asleep. Instead, if she's having trouble sleeping, she should get up, go to a different room, and do something quiet and boring (*not* watching an electronic screen like the TV, phone or iPad) until she feels sleepy. Then get back into bed and see if sleep overtakes her. Susannah's homework is to practice deep breathing three to four times a day for one minute at a time, at a rate of four breaths per minute, and to get out of bed if she is having trouble falling asleep.

Session 2

Session 2 begins with a review of the homework. Susannah reports that she practiced the deep breathing a few times a day. She likes it, and says it feels quite helpful, especially at night in bed when she is trying to relax and get to sleep. She has actually thought about incorporating it into a lesson plan for the kids she is student teaching. "It seems like it might be a great way to help them slow down and relax before tackling a difficult lesson." She only got out of bed one night when she had trouble winding down enough to sleep. She felt a little silly, but admitted that after sitting on the couch reading a magazine for about 20 minutes, she got sleepy, went back to bed, and fell right to sleep. She has been getting slightly better sleep and is feeling less exhausted overall, although she still feels quite fatigued and her joints still hurt. The therapist praises Susannah's use of these new skills, and agrees that teaching her students deep breathing is a great idea.

Susannah then confides that she still hasn't started taking the mesalamine. "I keep thinking I ought to be able to get this under control without needing medication," she says. The therapist strongly encourages Susannah to follow her doctor's advice on this score. She reminds Susannah that UC is an auto-immune disorder, and unless she can magically control her immune system in a way that other human beings can't, she really should take the medication. The therapist reiterates that mesalamine is considered the first line treatment for UC, and that for many people it will induce remission, both symptomatically, endoscopically and histologically. The therapist then proceeds to help Susannah identify her main goals of treatment. Susannah makes clear that she wants her life back. She wants to teach and get married and have a family of her own. The thing she fears most is that she won't be able to do these things, or that she will end up being a burden on her fiancé, Darius. Keeping these goals in mind, the therapist encourages Susannah to think through how taking the medication will be an important part of helping her achieve these goals. The healthier she is, the more likely she will be to be a successful teacher and an equal partner and parent. Susannah agrees to start taking the medication as prescribed.

At this point in the session, Susannah became quiet and tearful. The therapist probed gently to ask what she was thinking about. She shared that her relationship with Darius has been quite strained over the last month. She has been doing her best to soldier through and take care of things by herself because she doesn't want to depend on him or make him take care of her. She's also embarrassed about her symptoms and has tried to hide her frequent bathroom visits from him, preferring to cancel their plans if she feels like her gut is acting up. He has been alternately understanding and frustrated, especially when she cancels their plans at the last minute. "He's such a great guy – he deserves to be with someone who won't be sick all the time," she says.

The therapist asks Susannah more about her fiancé and the history of their relationship. It seems clear that Darius is, indeed, a great guy, who is committed to the relationship and very much wants to help her navigate the challenges of her illness. The therapist wonders whether perhaps Darius might actually be hurt that she is shutting him out. She asks Susannah to consider how she would feel if the situation were reversed – if Darius had been diagnosed with UC instead of her. Susannah sees instantly that she would want to know everything and would want to help in any way she could – "That's what a good marriage should be, you know, in sickness and in health. I would want to take care of him." The therapist gently points out that by shutting Darius out she is actually hurting their relationship and moving farther away from the trust and intimacy she wants. She agrees that even though it makes her nervous, she will talk to Darius about everything this weekend, and will be more honest with him moving forward. "I don't have to tell him about my bloody poop, though, do I? That seems like a real mood killer." The therapist laughingly agrees that that level of detail right off the bat might be a bit much, but that eventually in a good marriage, even bloody poop is something you can talk about.

Session 3

Susannah is pleased to announce at the beginning of the session that she has started taking the mesalamine as prescribed, and isn't noticing any weird side effects, but isn't feeling any better yet either. The therapist encourages Susannah to stick with it, and reminds her that it can take two to six weeks to start feeling better, so she shouldn't feel discouraged. The therapist also reminds Susannah that she needs to tell her gastroenterologist when she actually started taking it, so that they can accurately track her response to the medication. Susannah admits to some anxiety about doing this. "I'm afraid my doctor will yell at me or be disappointed or frustrated with me and think I'm a bad patient." The therapist reiterates how important it is to have open, honest communication with her gastroenterologist, and strongly encourages Susannah to use the online chart system to let her doctor know that she has now started the medication as prescribed.

Susannah also shares that she talked to Darius over the weekend. She was surprised at how hurt he had been by her efforts to "protect" him and not depend on him. "He said he *wants* me to be able to depend on him. Otherwise what's the point? I realized that shutting him out was a mistake. He felt like it meant I didn't trust him. Of course I trust him! I actually feel a lot closer to him now." The therapist praises Susannah warmly for being brave enough to talk to Darius honestly about her fears and her symptoms, and discusses how shame and secrecy are often the biggest burdens associated with GI disorders.

To further this point, the therapist asks what, if anything, Susannah has shared with her mentor teacher, the principal at the school, and her preceptor in her Master's program. Susannah looks at the therapist like the *therapist* is crazy and says, "Nothing! Why would I want to tell them what I'm dealing with? Okay, I get why Darius needed to know, but not my co-workers who are supervising and judging me and my work." The therapist guides Susannah to think through how stressful it is at work when she needs to use the bathroom but feels she can't step away from the class. She also acknowledges how embarrassed she is to have needed so many sick days over the last number of months. "I'm really worried they see me as unreliable or flaky." The therapist encourages Susannah to be honest with her co-workers. Susannah looks quite skeptical about this, but agrees to tell just her mentor teacher some of the basic facts of what she's been dealing with.

Session 4

Susannah is pleased to report that she told her mentor teacher about her UC and was pleasantly surprised that the senior teacher was not only sympathetic, she was pleased that Susannah had shared the truth with her. The senior teacher *had* been worried that Susannah wasn't really committed to teaching, despite her excellent work with the students when she was there, and was actually relieved to learn that Susannah had been coping with a specific medical issue and had simply been too embarrassed to tell her the truth. In a twist of fate, it turns out that the senior teacher's niece had been diagnosed with Crohn's Disease at age 16, and the teacher was familiar with IBDs and everything they entailed. Now that the teacher knows the truth, the two of them have come up with some strategies to manage it if Susannah does need to step out to use the bathroom. As a result, Susannah feels more confident about going in to teach even if her gut is acting up a bit in the morning, and she hasn't missed a day all week. She does admit, however, that she never eats breakfast or lunch on school days, to minimize the chances that she will need to run to the bathroom.

In light of the progress she has made, the therapist encourages Susannah to stop skipping breakfast and lunch. The therapist has Susannah consider the effects of hunger on her mood, concentration and energy. Indeed, she gets Susannah to acknowledge that when her pupils are irritable, reactive, distractible and tired it is often because they are hungry! Susannah agrees to try eating a small "safe" breakfast of soluble fiber rich oatmeal and a few blueberries or half a banana. With the "okay" from the gastroenterologist, Susannah also knows that she can take some anti-diarrheal medication on days when her gut is acting up. Overcoming her resistance to using any medication at all is somewhat challenging. Once again, the therapist reminds Susannah of her central goals and values. If the goal is to be an attentive, patient, effective teacher, then neither being hungry (and impatient and irritable) or needing to run to the rest room frequently are ideal. Using anti-diarrheal medication judiciously and appropriately can be an important part of managing her symptoms and allowing her to achieve her goals. Susannah admits that her doctor told her it was fine to use anti-diarrheal medication if she needed it, and that she will try it this week.

Session 5

Susannah is pleased to report that she ate breakfast every day this week, and did indeed feel more focused, had more energy, and felt quicker on her feet during her lessons. She used an anti-diarrheal medication three of the four days she was in the classroom and it did feel helpful. She actually didn't poop at all on day three, so she stopped taking the medication after that, and then had a normal bowel movement on the fifth day, followed by a return of some diarrhea thereafter. She notes that the burning pain seems to be lessening, and she hasn't noticed any mucous or blood in her stool all week. The therapist points out that this is good news, and that perhaps the mesalamine is starting to take effect. Susannah admits that she is feeling better and that getting through the day is starting to feel a bit more normal. She does admit that she still doesn't eat lunch on school days, partly because she is so busy and partly because she is afraid of bringing on symptoms. The therapist encourages her to try to fit in at least a small snack every day, pointing out that teaching is an intense job, and that all teachers need to learn to protect their own work-life balance and engage in appropriate self-care.

Susannah is still anxious about experiencing pain or feeling an urgent need to move her bowels during a class or during staff meetings, and she is very anxious about the upcoming parent-teacher conferences, which meet back to back for three hours without a break. While the senior teacher is primarily responsible for these, Susannah is expected to take part as well. Susannah is also anxious about an upcoming evaluation, in which her preceptor from her program will be observing her teach for an afternoon. The therapist encourages her to identify her catastrophic thoughts, and then replace them with more realistic, benign beliefs.

Session 6

Susannah reports that she got through the parent-teacher conferences successfully and notes that she was so busy and focused on what she needed to convey about each child that she actually didn't think about her gut at all. Her live evaluation went well. She felt somewhat crampy and uncomfortable that morning, so she did use some anti-diarrheal medication that day, but the actual teaching went well and she got through it with flying colors.

She also raises the issue that her cousin is getting married the following weekend, and she is supposed to be a bridesmaid. She is nervous about flying out of state and getting through the entire ceremony and reception. She has never been a nervous flyer in the past, but now the thought of being trapped in her seat on the airplane and then being around all her extended family (and all the strangers on her cousin's fiancé's side of the family) is making her feel like she should just cancel the whole trip. She is worried about being trapped in her seat on the plane and *needing* to use the toilet. She's also worried about drawing attention to herself if she feels sick during the wedding ceremony or the reception. She loves her aunt, uncle and cousin, and doesn't want to do anything to detract from their special day. "I don't want to make it about me – what if I get sick and ruin the whole day? I don't want them to hate me!"

The therapist reviews her fears about flying and about her extended family. Together they complete an imaginal exposure exercise in which the therapist walks her through an entire flight in imagination, including using the tiny airplane restroom, some turbulence, the seat belt sign being turned on, and the long wait to deplane at the gate. They also talk through the "worst-case scenario" for the wedding and think through how to talk to her cousin in advance. She is able to see that, like shutting Darius out early on, simply cancelling the trip and skipping the wedding is not the best option for anyone. She agrees that using anti-diarrheal medication is helpful, and that actually she is starting to feel better and better each week on the mesalamine, so perhaps the wedding trip won't be so difficult after all.

Session 7

Susannah skipped a week of treatment, since she was out of town at her cousin's wedding. She is pleased to report that the whole trip went off without a hitch. She was a little nervous standing in the security line at the airport on the trip out, but once she was on the plane she stayed occupied, reading a magazine, talking to Darius and even took a short nap. She didn't need to get up even once. The wedding itself was lovely, and she realizes how silly she's been thinking everyone would notice every little thing about her. She did excuse herself from the rehearsal dinner to go to the bathroom, but it was no big deal, and she doesn't think anyone even noticed. She got a little nervous about the drive from the ceremony to the reception. Darius was tasked with driving several elderly relatives and she rode with the other bridesmaid and a groomsman. She felt a few twinges of cramp on the drive, but she was able to breath and tell herself it was no big deal, and the cramps went away. Even if she had had to ask the driver to pull over at a gas station or convenience store so she could go to the bathroom, she realizes it would have been fine. She is thrilled that the flight and the wedding went off so successfully. Her confidence is growing, and she is starting to believe that she can live a normal, full life even with UC. Susannah and the therapist agree that she can wait two weeks for her next session.

Session 8

Susannah reports that, overall, she is pleased with how things are going. She is still anxious about what the future may hold, but she is feeling much more at peace and no longer believes that a teaching career and a life with Darius are out of reach.

Susannah shyly confides that now that she is feeling better, she and Darius are making love again. She admits that she had been feeling so ill, so unhappy with her body, and so terrified of experiencing incontinence and soiling the sheets and humiliating herself that she had stopped having sex with him months ago. She is feeling much more confident about the state of her bowels now. She did have a few concerning thoughts about how her body has changed. She is eating more regularly and has gained back some healthy weight in the time she's been in therapy, but she still feels terribly out of shape and flabby, and was worried that Darius would be totally turned off by her. Not surprisingly, Darius was an enthusiastic participant, and didn't seem the least bit concerned. He just stroked her face and told her how beautiful she was and how much he had missed her. She is thrilled to have that part of her life back.

Darius is now talking about taking a vacation together in the mountains. They used to hike together regularly, but since the onset of her UC she's been too worried about the proximity of bathrooms to risk being out in the wilderness. The therapist encourages her to start "small" by doing a day trip to a state park with public restroom facilities. The therapist then shared their own experiences with camping at relatively rough campsites. Susannah laughs and says the therapist may be willing to use stinky, gross out houses, but she is more civilized. Nicely appointed cabins with proper private bathrooms are more her style. But she is feeling much less anxious overall about the prospect of such a trip. She acknowledges that two months ago, it would have seemed impossible to even contemplate.

Towards the end of the session, the therapist reviews with Susannah everything she has learned, and confirms that her UC is now under far better control. She still has up to three loose bowel movements a day, but the burning pain and urgency have stopped, and she no longer sees any blood or mucous in her stool. Importantly, she is no longer afraid of experiencing incontinence. Moreover, she now understands that her catastrophic thoughts about what other people would think were distorted and unnecessarily negative. While she doesn't plan on telling everyone she meets that she has a "bloody poop" problem, she is much more comfortable sharing the basic outlines of UC with friends, extended family and co-workers. She is socializing again and has even started eating out – something she hadn't done in months. She is eating more regularly in general and has gained back some of the weight she had lost. She is still a little nervous about expanding her diet to include more soluble fiber and high FODMAP foods, but she is willing to give it a try. Most importantly, she no longer feels overwhelmed by the diagnosis or despairing about her future. She has a good working relationship with her gastroenterologist, and trusts her doctor to work with her collaboratively. She also understands the importance of being honest with her doctor and managing her care proactively to maximize her quality of life. With the therapist's reassurance that if she feels she needs more support in the future, she can always come back, Susannah decides to terminate therapy and tackle the rest of her issues on her own. She asks the therapist if she can have a hug, and thanks them fervently for "giving me hope for my life back."

Case 2: Mike

Session 1

Recall that Mike is a 54-year-old regional sales manager who has been living with Crohn's Disease since he was 14. He maintains a rigidly restrictive diet, and keeps his GI issues secret from everyone but his wife. He lives in fear of needing an ostomy, and doesn't understand why his gastroenterologist is telling him he's in remission when he is still experiencing so many GI symptoms, including abdominal pain, alternating diarrhea and constipation, gas and bloating. Mike arrives at his first session of therapy with a chip on his shoulder. He informs the therapist at the outset that he's not sure he believes in all this therapy mumbo-jumbo. He has a real disease – it's not all in his head – and he can't imagine how talking about any of it is going to make any difference. However, since his gastroenterologist strongly recommended the consult, and his wife is insisting he keep the appointment, he's decided to give this a shot.

Rather than diving in to taking a history, the therapist decides to address Mike's skepticism right off the bat. First, the therapist acknowledges that Mike is absolutely right – there *is* something truly wrong with his gut. Even if his Crohn's is mostly in remission, there is a good chance that he has developed central-enteric nervous system miscommunication, that his microbiome might be impoverished, and that stress is having a direct, biological effect on the functioning of the GI system. The therapist knows from the initial referral and consult with Mike's gastroenterologist that he is stable on Stelara dosed every eight weeks, and that she believes Mike has developed visceral hypersensitivity and secondary IBS. In order to help Mike understand visceral hypersensitivity, the therapist uses the example of phantom limb pain. Mike's father was a marine, and he knew many veterans growing up, so this explanation makes sense to him. Somewhat mollified, Mike asks how on earth talking is going to fix any of this. The therapist points out that "talking" affects how we think and what we believe – basic functions of the brain. By changing the way the brain interprets signals from the gut, and by changing the messages the brain itself is sending in response to threat and stress, Mike will actually be able to change the way his gut feels and works. Relaxing somewhat, Mike admits that that might make sense, and agrees to "go along" with what the therapist suggests "for now."

The therapist then takes a psychosocial and family history. Mike reports that his father was demanding, disciplined and somewhat harsh, but that Mike always respected him. Mike's father insisted that the house be kept spotless and would grow irate if things were out of place, or if Mike wore dirty shoes into the house, or broke some other rule. Mike learned to keep everything in his life clean and in perfect order. Although Mike's mother did most of the cooking, Mike's father always did the dishes when he was home, and had complicated rules for disinfecting the kitchen counters and the sink. Upon reflection, Mike realizes that some of his father's rules were extreme and probably didn't make sense. The therapist wonders out loud whether Mike's father might have had an obsessive-compulsive spectrum disorder. Mike bristles initially, but then admits that even for a military family, his dad seemed particularly rigid about cleaning, order and doing things the "right" way. "It was his way or the highway," Mike comments, "and God help you if you broke the rules." Upon further questioning, Mike describes his father's rules in more detail. Hands had to be washed with soap and scorching hot water for three full minutes after using the bathroom and before eating. Raw meat and eggs were kept strictly separate from all other food stuffs, and counters and cutting boards had to be disinfected with boiling water and bleach. If a utensil or a milk cap or jar lid fell on the floor, it had to be soaked in bleach for at least ten minutes and then washed. Mike reports that he himself has maintained some of these rules, and uses hand sanitizer after touching doorknobs, using public restrooms or shaking someone's hand. The therapist points out that there is a link between OCD (especially OCD with lots of cleaning compulsions) and auto-immune disorders. The therapist explains the hygiene hypothesis of auto-immune disorders and points out that Mike's compulsive sanitizing may actually be compromising his microbiome even now. In any case, Mike's stress levels (from his competitive job in which he has to "make his numbers" every month and every quarter and from keeping his GI issues secret) are clearly through the roof, and are making everything else harder to deal with. Mike admits that he's tightly wired "Type A" kind of guy, and that maybe learning to relax a little wouldn't kill him.

With this opening, the therapist teaches Mike deep diaphragmatic breathing. Mike is, as always, initially skeptical about this. The therapist is able to show Mike how his heart rate accelerates during an inhale and decelerates during a lengthy exhale, and assures him that those same parasympathetic processes will work on his gut as well. Mike agrees to try it over the course of the week. The therapist also sends him home with an OCD symptom checklist to complete, to ascertain the degree to which he might himself meet criteria for OCD.

Session 2

Mike begins session two by telling the therapist that deep breathing is helpful in the moment, when he's doing it, but hasn't had any effect at all on his overall symptoms. His alternating diarrhea, constipation, abdominal pain, and gas are as bad as ever. He did complete the OCD symptom checklist and says "I can't believe some of the crazy crap on this list. People really think this stuff?" He denied most obsessive symptom clusters (e.g. religious, sexual, violence and harm related themes), but did endorse perfectionistic checking and doubting, as well as a number of contamination fears and cleaning rituals. Although he says he's never had a particularly bad GI infection, he is terrified of contracting one, especially a C. diff. infection, that might make his symptoms worse. He thinks that would push him "right over the edge." His obsessions and compulsions are pervasive and time consuming enough that he meets criteria for mild to moderate OCD.

The therapist must now choose between initiating treatment for the OCD (which is undoubtedly adding to Mike's stress and exacerbating any underlying dysbiosis) versus continuing to address Mike's distressing GI symptoms directly. Working collaboratively, the therapist lays out the choice directly to Mike and asks him what he would rather work on first. Mike makes clear that although he is intrigued by this whole OCD thing and glad to hear treatment is possible, it's really the GI symptoms that are making him miserable. The therapist agrees to focus the next several sessions on GI symptom management but notes that it will make sense to return to the OCD relatively soon.

The rest of the session is spent exploring Mike's catastrophic beliefs and language about his GI symptoms. He shares the fear that his whole GI system will just "rot from the inside out" and confides that when he is experiencing GI pain he gets so worried about it that he can't focus on anything else. He did undergo a surgical resection about five years ago that was deemed a success. His last colonoscopy six months ago showed some minor inflammation around the anastomosis, but confirmed that otherwise his intestinal tissues look good. A capsule endoscopy also showed no signs of ulcerations or new strictures in the upper and middle small intestine. Nevertheless, he is terrified that he will experience further inflammation, ulcerations, strictures or a fistula and will end up with a permanent ostomy as his only option. If he experiences any abdominal pain during the day, he thinks to himself, "Oh no – here we go again. My Crohn's is out of control. The darn medication isn't working anymore. Now what am I going to do?" The therapist then works with him on combating his catastrophic beliefs that his GI system will "rot" and that he cannot have a productive or enjoyable day if he is experiencing GI discomfort. The therapist also cites some of the data on quality of life in ostomates and suggests that while there is currently no reason to believe that Mike will need one, his worst-case scenario of needing an ostomy would almost certainly not be as bad he fears. The therapist encourages Mike to continue with deep breathing, and to reframe his GI symptoms as uncomfortable, but not dangerous or catastrophic.

Session 3

Mike reports he is still very bothered by GI symptoms, especially constipation. At the time of the session, he notes that he hasn't defecated in three days. "If I could just go like a normal person my life would be fine." The therapist reviews his medications and diet. He takes colestipol on a rigid schedule to counteract any bile acid malabsorption from the resection. The therapist encourages him to consider adjusting the dose, or even skipping a day when he is constipated. His diet is also quite low in fiber, secondary to his anxiety about experiencing an obstruction or "over taxing" his intestines, so the therapist gently encourages him to add more soluble fiber and to drink more water. Mike usually has a cup of hot water for breakfast. The therapist encourages him to try oatmeal or granola with fruit. Mike always thought oatmeal was "binding" and is interested to learn about the distinction between insoluble and soluble fiber. He is still resistant to the notion that simply relabeling his current symptoms as "uncomfortable sensations" rather than pain will do any good. "You can call it whatever you want, but I know it's pain," he insists.

The therapist then asks Mike about his job. It is demanding, fast paced, and his work is often carefully scrutinized by his managers and the VP of the company. Mike notes that he usually double- and triple-checks everything he does to ensure accuracy. He notes that the turnover rate in the profession is very high and that one of colleagues (another regional manager) recently retired early after experiencing a mild heart attack. When the therapist asks if he would ever consider changing careers, he says no. He makes excellent money. He also notes that when he is healthy, he loves the intensity and the competitive nature of the job. "When my numbers are good, I'm the best in the business," he says. It's just now that his gut is acting up it makes it hard to focus and makes him doubt himself. He worries that he will make a mistake, or fail to follow-up on something important, and could cost his company a major contract worth millions of dollars. He has always checked his work multiple times, but now he's rarely satisfied. He has even started checking emails he sends multiple times to be sure there are no typos or errors in them. The therapist points out that his OCD *seems* to serve him well at times. When he is at the top of his game, he can triple-check everything (as his OCD demands) and be assured that he is doing a good job. But when he isn't feeling well, the OCD makes him especially doubtful that he has made a mistake. This is extremely anxiety provoking and leads to his feeling overwhelmed at work. At this point, Mike actually starts to become tearful. "I really want to be excellent at my job – the best," he says. "I just don't know if I can keep doing it through all this pain." The therapist points out the irony that Mike's intensity and distress are leading him to consider taking a leave from work that is lucrative and that he loves and suggests that targeting the OCD and his anxiety about his GI symptoms may well enable him to function effectively again. Mike expresses hope that that would work. For homework, the therapist encourages Mike to alter his diet to include more soluble fiber (and water), to dose the colestipol more flexibly and to start keeping track of how often he doubts his work and double and triple-checks himself.

Session 4

Mike starts the session by announcing that he has defecated every day this week but once, hasn't had any diarrhea, and that oatmeal is fantastic. The therapist is pleased that Mike is feeling better but cautions him against concluding that oatmeal was the "magic bullet." Eating breakfast, especially with some soluble fiber, probably helps, the therapist explains, but it would be good to mix it up and try to expand his diet to include other foods as well. Mike *is* feeling better, but is still concerned about frequent abdominal pain, and still feels very overwhelmed at work. One morning he didn't feel the urge to defecate until he got to work. Too embarrassed to use the men's room on his floor (where his managers and peers might hear and smell the results), he made a point of going down two floors to another department entirely and used the rest room there. The therapist takes this opportunity to talk about social anxiety and how fear of embarrassment can make life more difficult for people with GI disorders. The therapist asks if his co-workers ever defecate in the bathroom. Mike admits that they do and the therapist encourages Mike to just use the restroom on his floor in the future. The therapist also discusses experiential avoidance more generally and points out that all of his efforts to avoid discomfort and embarrassment have actually made his problems worse. The therapist lists the many things Mike does to avoid anxiety around contamination and the possibility of making mistakes, to avoid embarrassment, to avoid work when his gut is uncomfortable and to avoid visceral sensations all together. "How's that workin' for ya?" the therapist asks. Mike admits that his quality of life and productivity have been getting worse and worse over the last few years, and that it may be time to try a new strategy.

The therapist now introduces the notion of exposure therapy, which will be helpful for both OCD and for reducing visceral hypersensitivity. The therapist has a small mandarin orange on their desk, which they peel and divide into multiple sections. The therapist asks Mike how uncomfortable it would make him to eat a piece of orange that had touched the coffee table, or the carpeted floor, or his shoe. He looks at the therapist as if they are crazy. "Who in their right mind would eat something off a shoe?" he asks. "Well, I would," the therapist replies, "if it will help you overcome your OCD. I will never ask you to do anything I wouldn't do." The therapist places a segment of orange on the top of their shoe and encourages Mike to eat a piece of orange that has touched the table, then a piece that has touched the arm of the couch. This makes him extremely uncomfortable, but he is willing to try it. The therapist then eats a piece of orange that has been on the carpet, and finally eats the piece that has been resting on their shoe. Mike sits with the discomfort and says, "If I get really sick tonight I'll know who to blame!" The therapist praises his courage and willingness to engage in exposure and moves the conversation on to homework. Mike agrees to use the bathroom on his floor at work, to go to work even if he isn't feeling well, and to try to stop washing his hands so frequently and to throw out the hand sanitizer. At the end of the session, the therapist asks how anxious he is feeling about having eaten the orange slices. He admits that he had actually stopped thinking about it, and is no longer uncomfortable with it.

Session 5

Mike returns for session five very agitated and distressed. He says he was doing fine until two days ago, at which point he began to experience abdominal distention and bloating at work one afternoon. He left work early and went home, focusing more and more on the sensations in his gut, feeling like he needed to defecate, but couldn't. He spent the evening sitting on the toilet getting more and more frustrated and anxious and feeling worse and worse. It got so bad, he convinced his wife to take him to the ER at around 11 pm, as he was convinced he had developed a small bowel obstruction. After an imaging study revealed simple constipation, the ER doctor suggested he try Miralax and sent him home with 1 mg of alprazolam to help him sleep. He stayed home the next day as well. Mike is exhausted and angry. "I thought this was supposed to be helping me, but it's just as bad as ever!" The therapist empathizes with his distress and says, "It sounds like you were really scared and at your wits end that night." "Yes," Mike replies. "I really thought I might die. It was terrifying." The therapist then guides Mike to think through how his vivid catastrophic thoughts that night led to an increase of cramping, pain and spasms in his pelvic floor muscles. The therapist reminds Mike about the effects of sympathetic arousal on the entire GI system and points out that catastrophizing almost certainly exacerbated the pain and panic and made the problem much worse. Exhaustion and sleep deprivation also didn't help. Mike is also angry at the ER doctor, whom he felt was dismissive and rude. "He treated me like I was crazy," Mike complains. "I have Crohn's Disease, for God's sake. It's real. It could kill me someday." The therapist gently guides Mike to consider the possibility that the ER doctor was also tired and busy and may have been brusque and unsympathetic because they had so many other patients to take care of. The therapist also encourages Mike to consider that he was engaging in catastrophic distortions about his symptoms, which made his pain worse. He does have Crohn's Disease, but all the evidence is that it's under good medical control at the moment. He was constipated and gassy, which was definitely uncomfortable, but not dangerous in any way. Had he simply eaten some oatmeal or taken some Metamucil, drunk his hot water, and gone to work, his day probably would have gone much better.

The therapist encourages Mike to try to go to work every day and to remind himself that constipation is *uncomfortable and annoying* but not dangerous. The therapist also asks Mike about his exercise regimen and explains that exercise is one of the best ways to burn off stress and to get the GI system moving. Mike was an active, athletic kid before he got sick and tells the therapist that he used to enjoy running and playing tennis when he was younger, but he feels like the Crohn's has sapped his energy so much over the last 20 years that he has felt too worn down to work out. The therapist encourages Mike to start exercising again by going for a brisk walk or jog several times a week and maybe hitting some balls with his wife at the tennis club. Mike is skeptical (as always) that going for a walk will do any good ("Won't it just make me more tired?") but reluctantly agrees to start including some mild exercise in his week.

Session 6

Mike reports feeling much better this week. He has defecated most days, mostly formed stool, and is trying hard not to catastrophize or panic on mornings when he doesn't defecate or days when he has several loose bowel movements. He has gone to work every day. He did use the restroom on his floor once, although he wasn't happy about it. He acknowledges that if someone else is defecating, it bothers him, and he doesn't like the smell. He is always quick to leave the room before the other person emerges from their stall in order to save them both from embarrassment. The therapist praises Mike for the strides he is making and admits that no one "likes" the smell of poop. However, the therapist encourages Mike to stay in the bathroom long enough to make eye contact and engage in casual banter with other people from time to time. Mike also notes that he went on brisk walks twice and even tried jogging for a few miles, although he and his wife haven't been to the tennis club yet. He is dismayed and embarrassed about how out of shape he is. The therapist praises Mike for starting to exercise again and reminds him to take it slow. Mike says that although he was frustrated with how out of shape he is, he did feel calmer and more centered after each walk.

The therapist then asks him about hand washing, hand sanitizing, and use of antiseptic and antibacterial products around the house. Mike admits that it is hard for him to change old habits, but that he understands why it might be important. "We never used to have hand sanitizer," he admits. "I followed Dad's rules at home, but when I was with my friends we just ate without washing our hands and the other guys never got sick." This insight helps him commit to exposing himself to more things without engaging in cleaning compulsions. In session, he agrees to put his hands on the floor, and then rub them on his clothes. The therapist models rubbing their hand on the bottom of their shoe and then touching their hair and face. Not to be outdone, Mike takes off one shoe and, with a grimace, touches the sole to his cheek. "There, you happy?" he asks the therapist with mock belligerence. For homework, Mike agrees to continue exposing himself to possible "contamination" at home. He notes that if he eats something off the floor, his wife will be shocked but thrilled. She has always thought his rules about cleanliness were excessive.

Session 7

Mike continues to make good progress with both his contamination focused OCD symptoms and his catastrophizing about his GI symptoms. However, he is still bothered by his GI symptoms at work and is now fixated on the possibility that he will have to leave a meeting to go the bathroom. He has never confided in anyone at work about his difficulties and is appalled when the therapist suggests sharing that he has chronic GI issues with a few key people. "Are you kidding?" he asks. "I would never talk about this stuff at work – it's disgusting and pathetic. I don't want people pitying me or worse thinking I'm off my rocker. You show weakness in my line of work, and your head is on the chopping block." The therapist helps Mike unpack all the negative, catastrophic distortions and beliefs embedded in this. GI problems do not make a person "disgusting and pathetic" or "off their rocker." Acknowledging a health problem is unlikely to get him fired. Moreover, Mike need not frame it in a way that evokes pity or makes him look weak. Rather, the therapist suggests that Mike say simply, "Hey, just wanted to let you know I've got some chronic GI issues. I'm handling it and getting it treated, but I may need to excuse myself from meetings every so often to hit the men's room." Mike admits that when it is framed that way, it doesn't sound so bad, and agrees to tell his direct manager.

The therapist also urges Mike to have a conversation with his children about his GI issues. Mike acknowledges that keeping his Crohn's Disease secret from his kids has caused a good deal of tension and distance in his relationship with them. "Their mom does everything for them. I would love to go to their games or meets when I'm in town. I just don't want to embarrass them by needing to go to the bathroom all the time. Plus some of those tournaments and venues are crazy. There might be just a few porta potties five fields away. What if I couldn't get there?" The therapist helps Mike think through how all this secrecy has compromised his relationship with his kids, and how his efforts to spare them (and himself) embarrassment may have led them to believe that he doesn't *want* to be involved in their lives. They spend some time role playing how the conversation might go. Initially, the therapist models what Mike could say to them. "Well, it doesn't sound so bad when you say it," Mike admits. Then Mike practices it until he feels comfortable. "My wife will be thrilled," he says. "She already thinks you walk on water. If I can start driving the kids to some of their activities, she'll want to nominate you for sainthood." The therapist points out that the real benefit will be increased closeness with his kids. He'll be modeling resilience and coping and the kids will know how important they are to him and how much he loves them.

Session 8

Mike reports that he did tell his direct manager about his Crohn's Disease as planned. His manager was shocked to learn that Mike had a chronic disease he'd been living with for years. This provided Mike with some useful feedback. He always thought his bathroom issues and occasional absences from work or meetings were incredibly noticeable and a real concern to his boss. He was both surprised and relieved to discover that his issues really weren't all that obvious. If anything, Mike's boss had been concerned that Mike was actually using his sick days to interview at other firms. The manager was pleased that Mike had let him know, and assured Mike that he was a valued member of the team and one of their top performers. He even offered to let Mike work remotely a day or two a week if that would help. While the therapist is pleased the experience of confiding in his manager went so well, they discourage Mike from taking up the offer to work remotely for now. It is more important to get himself into the office on a regular basis. Ironically, now that Mike knows it wouldn't be a big deal to step out of a meeting, he has not felt the urge to do so.

Mike's conversation with his children also went well, although not the way he expected. In the mirror image of the conversation with his boss, his kids said they always knew he had something going on, but had been afraid to ask about it because they thought it would make him mad. Mike actually grew a little tearful in relating this story. "I never want my kids to be afraid of me," he said. "I was kind of afraid of my dad. I never felt like I could tell him stuff. Even when I got sick in high school I felt like he just wanted me to soldier on and not complain. He wasn't the most sympathetic guy on the planet. I guess I've been trying to be tough and strong like him. But I want my kids to know that they can talk to me about anything. I guess trying to keep this whole Crohn's Disease thing secret from them backfired big time." The therapist praises Mike warmly for having the conversation with his kids, and for his insights about how his own childhood experiences colored his view of how he was "supposed" to manage his disease. The therapist points out that Mike can be a model for his kids of resilience and effective coping with adversity. The therapist also asks Mike to imagine a time when he and his family can be open with one another and even joke about his GI issues and OCD. Mike is thoughtful for a moment, and points out that he has wondered if his son might have some mild OCD as well. He describes some of his son's behavior, and the therapist agrees it is a possibility, and offers him a referral to a colleague who specializes in pediatric OCD. "Better to nip it in the bud, I guess," Mike says.

Overall, Mike's GI symptoms are bothering him much less and he is less prone to catastrophizing and thinking about worst-case scenarios. He is no longer convinced that his Crohn's is actively progressing or that his gut is going to "rot" from the inside, and now believes his test results and the reassurance of his doctor. He has accepted that stress was exacerbating his symptoms and making them much worse, and that he had (understandably) developed visceral hypersensitivity after years of living with a chronic GI disease. He still has work to do on his OCD and may well continue in therapy for several more months to bring that under better control, but overall he is pleased with his progress, and admits that "all this talking" did somehow make his gut feel better and has improved his quality of life, both at work and with his family

Final Thoughts

Susannah and Mike are representative cases of how a cognitive-behavioral therapist might work with a patient with an IBD. In both cases, the therapist conferred with the gastroenterologist at least once, and facilitated a more honest and collaborative relationship between the patient and their doctor. It is noteworthy that Susannah had no psychiatric diagnoses prior to onset of the UC, and that her distress was acute and best characterized as an Adjustment Disorder. Mike, on the other hand, had suffered from obsessive-compulsive disorder for many years. In both cases, addressing the cognitive distortions, emotional distress, family system and work-related issues brought about significant relief and dramatically improved their quality of life and their ability to *cope with Crohn's and colitis*. My hope is that this book will help others achieve the same good outcomes.

Acknowledgments

First and foremost, I would like to acknowledge the specific undergraduate students who have worked in my lab and made my research in this area possible, and without whom this treatment program and this book would not exist.

Lauren Rodriguez was the first student to suggest that I really ought to expand both my research and my clinical work from my focus on IBS to include patients with IBD. Her warmth, enthusiasm for the project and confidence that it was doable convinced me to try.

Enitan Marcelle joined forces with Lauren Rodriguez to test out a modularized version of the new treatment in a pilot trial during which we learned a lot from the patients who participated and refined the treatment still more. Her deep intelligence, quiet intensity and good humor helped keep me motivated and between them we finished the trial and got the paper published against what felt like long odds.

Lauren Smith spent a full year helping me turn the modularized treatment into a standalone self-help book. She brought a deft touch and excellent writing skills, and in particular helped draft the chapter on living with an ostomy. She was also instrumental in helping me get feedback on the book from relevant stakeholders. She is incisive, a quick study, and *much* warmer than she thinks she is.

Mary Keenan and Michael Accardo helped shepherd the IRB protocol for the next clinical trial, and developed what was *supposed* to be a placebo control "book" to compare this book to. Carefully curated and compiled from existing resources available on the web, they kept insisting that it might actually be helpful to patients, and I kept saying "It better not be!" They were right, and I was humbled, though I'm pleased to report that this book was significantly *more* helpful.

Paddy Loftus spent the summer after his freshman year attending CCF support groups and meeting with gastroenterologists with me, and then took over the management of the clinical trial of this book with energy, creativity, intellectual rigor and phenomenal interpersonal skills. I was truly fortunate that he landed in my lab and still can't believe how much he accomplished in such a short amount of time.

Lauren Cohen (I seem to have a lot of students named Lauren) helped Paddy with recruitment and data cleaning and came up with a way to measure compliance that was truly helpful. Her quiet, reliable, thoughtful approach to both patient care and analytical strategies was indispensable.

DOI: 10.4324/9781003057635-17

The paper we published from the clinical trial was a group effort that was a number of years in the making.

I could never do everything I do without these phenomenal students. I am incredibly proud of all of them. Lauren R., Enitan, Lauren S., Mary, Michael and Paddy are all pursuing or have already obtained PhDs in psychology. Lauren C. is pursuing an MPH in public health and epidemiology. We should all count ourselves lucky that such bright, thoughtful, caring, creative young professionals are in the world and will be the next generation of leading clinical scientists and therapists.

Thanks also to Mark Osterman, MD, MSCE, a gastroenterologist and IBD specialist who believed in my work, helped me recruit patients for our trial, and taught me a lot about the medical side of inflammatory bowel diseases. Any errors or misrepresentations of those issues are mine alone.

I owe an enormous debt and deep gratitude to the incomparable Dr. Aaron T. Beck, the inventor of Cognitive Therapy, and one of my early mentors in clinical psychology. Little did I know when I moved to Philadelphia for graduate school that I would have the privilege of learning directly from one of the truly great minds (and hearts) of all time. Dr. Beck is one of the most brilliant, creative and generous mentors in the world. His enthusiasm and support for my work over the years has meant the world to me. I count myself incredibly fortunate to have studied with him.

Thanks to my colleagues in the Department of Psychology at the University of Pennsylvania, including Dianne Chambless, Rob DeRubeis, Sara Jaffee and Ayelet Ruscio, model clinical scientists all, who create a supportive atmosphere for the difficult work we all do and provide me with much needed consults, advice, and encouragement. Thanks also to folks who have served as Chair of the department during my time at Penn, including Robert Seyfarth, Dave Brainard, Sharon Thompson-Schill and Dan Swingley. Their collective vision and flexibility have given me the freedom to see my patients and to pursue the research I love.

I owe a (very belated, but none less heartfelt) thanks to Dr. Jodi Mindell, colleague, neighbor and friend extraordinaire who taught me how to write a book proposal and made possible the leap from academic writing to writing for a broader audience.

Thanks to all the folks at Routledge/Taylor and Francis who thought this book was a good bet, and were extraordinarily patient with me when the COVID pandemic derailed my efforts to get the MS to them in a timely way.

Thanks to all three of my kids for keeping me on my toes – to Ian for his enthusiasm and willingness to push me when I'm stuck, to Noah for his quiet grounding, support and deft touch when I'm distressed, and to Anna Rose, the only one still at home, who can blow me away with her nuanced perspective on social justice and schools me on the use of punctuation in text messages (just don't). They all challenge me with new ideas, delight me with their talents and accomplishments and fill me with pride at what lovely, mature, responsible and kind people they have all turned out to be.

Thanks to my parents, Irene Winter and Robert Hunt, for continuing to provide guidance, advice, encouragement and support. At 81 and 87, they both keep telling me they're going to retire from scholarship sometime soon. I'll believe it when I see it. I count myself doubly blessed that I still have them as role models both personally and professionally.

And finally, thanks as always to my beloved husband, Garth Isaak. Marrying you was by far the smartest thing I've ever done. That fortune I got the first time we ate at a Chinese restaurant together was truly prescient. In the eyes of love, even scars can look like dimples. I *still* can't believe how lucky I am.

References

Belling, R., Woods, L. & McLaren, S. (2008). Stakeholder perceptions of specialist Inflammatory Bowel Disease nurses' role and personal attributes. *International Journal of Nursing Practice*, 14(1), 67–73. doi:10.1111/j.1440-172X.2007.00661.x.

Craven, M.R., Quinton, S. & Taft, T.H. (2018). Inflammatory bowel disease patient experiences with psychotherapy in the community. *Journal of Clinical Psychology in Medical Settings*. doi:10.1007/s1088-0-018-9576-9575.

Dainty, A., Hunt, M., Holtham, E., Kinsella, P., Timmons, S., Fox, M. & Callaghan, P., (2017). An embedded mixed methods feasibility study evaluating the use of low-intensity, nurse-delivered Cognitive Behavioural Therapy for the treatment of Irritable Bowel Syndrome. *Gastrointestinal Nursing*, 15(9), 39–49. doi:10.12968/gasn.2017.15.9.39.

Evertsz', F.B., Bockting, C.L., Stokkers, P.C., Hinnen, C., Sanderman, R. & Sprangers, M. A. (2012). The effectiveness of cognitive behavioral therapy on the quality of life of patients with inflammatory bowel disease: multi-center design and study protocol (KL!C- study). *BMC Psychiatry*. doi:10.1186/1471-1244-12-227.

Evertsz', F.B., Thijssens, N., Stokkers, P., Grootenhuis, M., Bockting, C., Nieuwkerk, P. & Sprangers, M. (2012). Do inflammatory bowel disease patients with anxiety and depressive symptoms receive the care they need? *Journal of Crohn's and Colitis*, 6(1), 68–76. doi:10.1016/j.crohn s.2011.07.006.

Häuser, W., Moser, G., Klose, P. & Miocka-Walus, A. (2014). Psychosocial issues in evidence-based guidelines on inflammatory bowel diseases: A review. *World Journal of Gastroenterology*, 20, 3663–3671.

Mayberry, M.K. & Mayberry, J.F. (2003). The status of nurse practitioners in gastroenterology. *Clinical Medicine*, 3(1), 37–41. doi:10.7861/clinmedicine.3-1-37.

Sajadinejad, M.S., Asgari, K., Molavi, H., Kalantari, M. & Adibi, P. (2012). Psychological issues in inflammatory bowel disease: an overview. *Gastroenterology Research and Practice*, 106502. doi:10.1155/2012/106502.

Szigethy, E.M., Allen, J.I., Reiss, M., Cohen, W., Perera, L.P., Brillstein, L., … Regueiro, M. D. (2017). The impact of mental and psychosocial factors on the care of patients with inflammatory bowel disease. *Clinical Gastroenterology and Hepatology*, 15, 986–997.

Index